FREE FOODS

FREE

FOODS

Guilt-free food for
healthy appetites

EBURY
PRESS

First published in 2005

1 3 5 7 9 10 8 6 4 2

First published by Ebury Press
Random House, 20 Vauxhall Bridge Road,
London SW1V 2SA

Random House Australia (Pty) Limited
20 Alfred Street, Milsons Point, Sydney,
New South Wales 2061, Australia

Random House New Zealand Limited
18 Poland Road, Glenfield, Auckland 10,
New Zealand

Random House South Africa (Pty) Limited
Endulini, 5a Jubilee Road, Parktown 2193,
South Africa

The Random House Group Limited
Reg. No. 954009

www.randomhouse.co.uk

A CIP catalogue record for this book is available
from the British Library

ISBN 0 09 1901650

Editor: Emma Callery
Recipes created by Sunil Vijayakar
Design: Roger Hammond @ Blue Gum

Food photography: Jon Whitaker
Food stylist: Sunil Vijayakar
Prop stylist: Rachel Jukes

For Slimming World
Founder and Chairman: Margaret Miles-Bramwell
Managing Director: Caryl Richards
Project co-ordinator: Allison Brentnall
Text by Christine Michael Whelan

Printed and bound in China by C&C Offset
Printing Co., Ltd

SLIMMING WORLD

Founded in 1969 by Margaret Miles-Bramwell, Slimming World is the UK's most advanced slimming organisation. It currently manages thousands of groups across the country, with over 250,000 members attending every month, and another 15,000 attending free as successful target members. Each week, around 2,000 members reach their personal target weight. Slimming World's unique approach to weight loss is an extraordinary success story.

COOKERY NOTES

■ Both metric and imperial measures are given for the recipes.
Follow either set of measures as they are not interchangeable.

■ All spoon measures are level: 1 tsp = 5ml spoon, 1 tbsp = 15ml spoon.

■ Ovens should be preheated to the specified temperature.
Grills should also be preheated.

■ Use large eggs unless otherwise specified.

■ Note that some of the recipes contain lightly cooked eggs. Avoid serving these to anyone who is pregnant or in a vulnerable health group, because of the small risk of salmonella infection.

■ Always use fresh herbs, unless dried herbs are suggested in the recipe.

■ Use freshly ground black pepper and sea salt unless otherwise specified.

CONTENTS

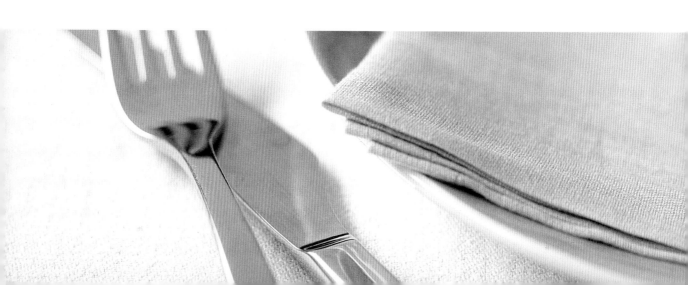

Dear Reader

A VERY WARM WELCOME TO *FREE FOODS*! As Slimming World's Founder and Chairman I'm so excited that from all the glossy recipe books on the shelves – so many it can be hard to know where to start – you've chosen this one. In this stunning collection of recipes, you'll find inspiring ideas for delicious meals designed with modern lifestyles in mind – quick, easy and healthy.

Yet *Free Foods* offers you so much more! The title comes from Free Food, the powerhouse of Slimming World's revolutionary Food Optimising system, which has helped hundreds of thousands of men and women to lose weight effectively and to maintain a healthy weight successfully. Free Food is the key that breaks you out of the 'diet trap' of feeling guilty, deprived or out of control around food and, furthermore, it opens the door to a whole new way of eating and managing your weight that's enjoyable, empowering and, above all, liberating.

The recipes in this collection will help you explore Free Food to the full, and to discover just how you can satisfy your appetite by eating delicious foods, whenever or wherever you like, and still lose weight. That's the power of Free Food; it's amazingly simple, and simply amazing.

Yet there's even more to Food Optimising than Free Food, and there's even more to Slimming World than Food Optimising. For over 35 years it's been my personal life goal to help slimmers escape the misery of excess weight, and with that goal constantly in sight, Slimming World has evolved into a uniquely powerful and effective support system for anyone who wants to lose weight and maintain a healthy weight for life.

As someone for whom weight has always been a personal issue, I believe passionately that group support, shared experience and unconditional approval are the key elements that help slimmers conquer their fears, confront their demons and overcome difficulties in a way that exceeds not just their expectations but their dreams. That warmth and support are what the 250,000 members who attend Slimming World experience in their groups every week provide, with simply amazing results.

In this book we can only offer you a brief insight into everything that Slimming World has to offer. We hope that the recipes will capture your imagination and show you just how generous, refreshing and slimmer-friendly a weight-loss system can be.

And if you are someone who loves food but thought you'd never find a way of managing your weight that fits in with your lifestyle – join the club! We'd love to welcome you in person and have the privilege of helping you on your own journey to freedom. Together, we can do it!

This book can change your life and it comes to you as always, with love.

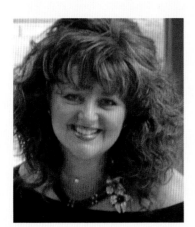

Margaret Miles-Bramwell
Founder and Chairman

FOOD OPTIMISING

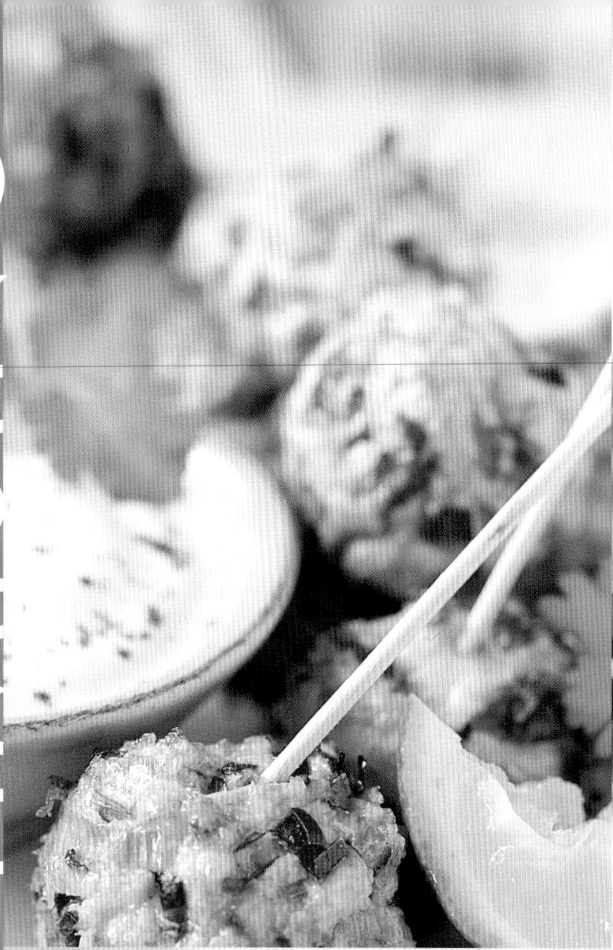

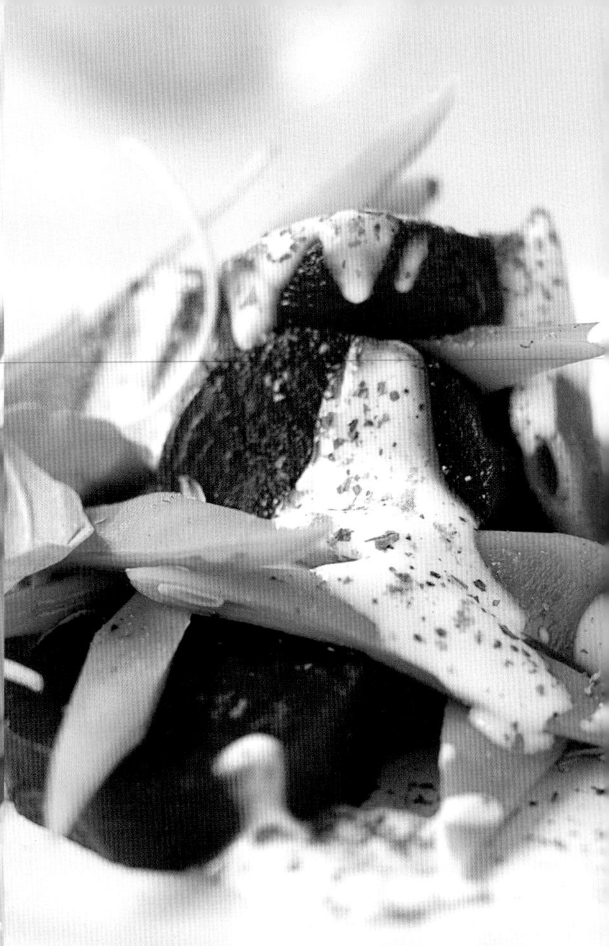

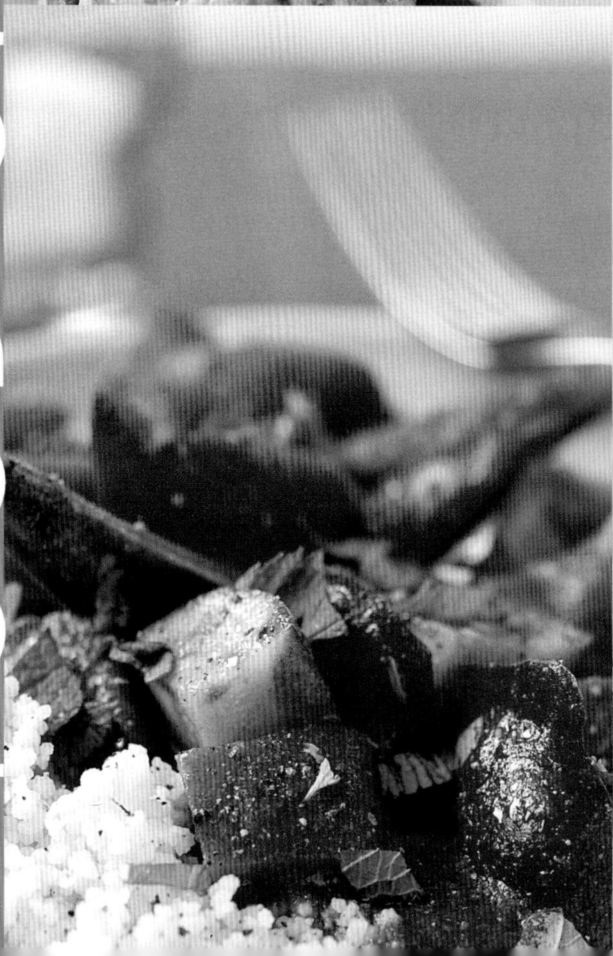

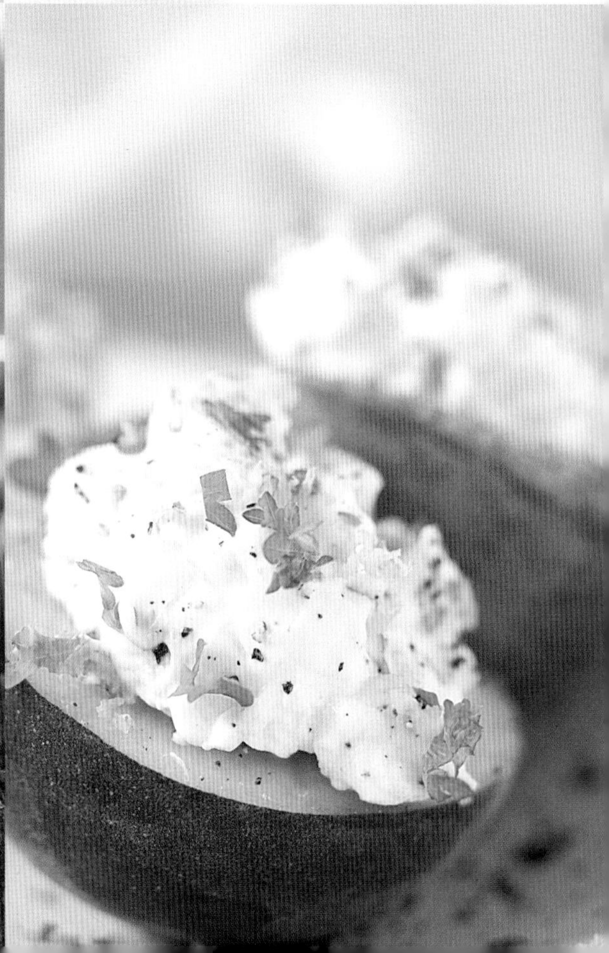

FREE TO ENJOY

COOKERY BOOKS HAVE come a long way since the first published collections of 'receipts', with their closely typed lists of instructions and no pictures. Today we love recipe books because they celebrate the joys of food; looking at the glossy colour photographs and reading the tempting descriptions are all part of the highly enjoyable process of planning, preparing and eating a meal.

A quick look through this book is all you need to see that Free Foods is every bit as glossy and tempting as anything a celebrity chef has to offer – with the bonus that our recipes are designed for everyday cooking in ordinary kitchens, not to look good in restaurants or TV studios.

But the real 'star quality' of these recipes is that they have all been devised in line with Food Optimising – Slimming World's unique and sophisticated way of eating healthily and losing weight. As we hope you will discover for yourself, Food Optimising makes it easy for you to reach the weight you want to be – and stay there – without ever going hungry, feeling guilty or compromising on your love of good food.

You might think that's a big claim to make. But with over 35 years' experience of helping people to free themselves from the burden of being overweight, Slimming World has unbeatable expertise, a deep understanding and, above all, an unquenchable passion to help members achieve their weight-loss goals and see their dreams of a healthy, happy lifestyle become reality.

The key to our confidence can be found in the title of this book: *Free Foods*. The title comes from Free Food, which is the powerhouse of Slimming World's Food Optimising system.

THE VALUE OF FREE FOOD

As you will find as you read this brief introduction, Free Food is simply amazing. First, it is simple because by satisfying your appetite on Free Food you can eat as much as you like of wholesome, fresh, everyday foods – as much as you like! – without having to weigh, measure, count or follow any of the boring rules or petty restrictions that you might normally associate with a weight-loss plan. Second, it is amazing because Free Food turns the conventional wisdom about dieting on its head, with spectacular results. Hundreds of thousands of slimmers have found that at Slimming World, the

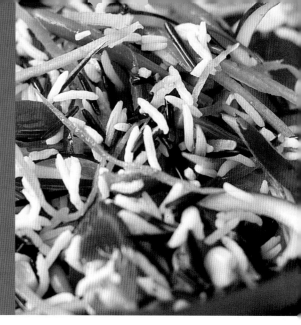

■ Instead of asking you to eat less, **Free Food** encourages you to eat more!

■ Instead of dictating what you eat, **Free Food** offers you more choice than you ever thought possible!

■ Instead of laying down the law on when or how you eat, **Free Food** is the way to ensure that your eating plan fits into your life, not the other way round!

simply amazing power of Free Food has enabled them to achieve weight losses that they could never have dreamed of – even if they had tried many times before, and even if they had long since convinced themselves that 'diets didn't work' for them.

In devising the recipes for this new collection, our aim is to excite, inspire and thrill you with the possibilities of Free Food. If you are already a Slimming World member, you'll find dozens of new ideas to liven up your menus and fuel your imagination with the versatility and variety that Free Food has to offer. And if this is the first time you have read about Slimming World, we're sure you'll be intrigued and delighted to see just how delicious and satisfying healthy eating can be.

TAKE CONTROL

It may be that you have no trouble maintaining your weight, but just love trying out new foods and new dishes to share with friends and family. If you're in that happy position, you will enjoy all the tasty, filling, great-looking recipes in this book. But if weight is an issue for you, and if you have ever despaired of finding a way of eating that works with your lifestyle, not against it, *Free Foods* offers far more: it offers you the opportunity to discover a new approach to managing your weight that you will find refreshing, enjoyable and, above all, liberating.

At Slimming World, we fervently believe that slimmers deserve to feel free around food: free to enjoy the food choices they make and to take real pleasure in eating, instead of feeling trapped, guilty or out of control. Free Food will show you how to take back that control, and exercise your power of

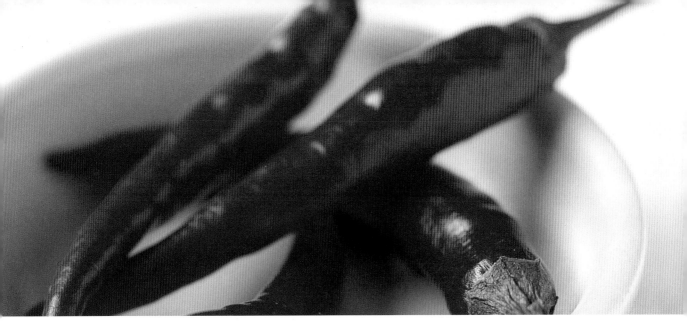

choice – and in the most remarkable of ways! On one level, for example, if the thought of spending time around food makes you anxious about cooking and eating too much, Free Food can put the fun back into your kitchen. With Free Food, you can make fantastic meals without feeling guilty about licking the bowl, tasting as you go or finishing off the leftovers!

And if you worry that cooking 'diet meals' means lots of time and effort spent making tiny portions of dishes that the family won't touch, think again! *Free Foods* features dozens of filling, everyday meals that will quickly become firm favourites with both your family and friends. And when they see just how high you pile your plate, no one will believe you're slimming – not even you, as the resident chef!

Above all, the recipes in this book harness the power of Free Food to help you experience just how flexible, enjoyable and generous Food Optimising is. But there is far more to Food Optimising than Free Food – and there is far more to Slimming World than Food Optimising!

THE POWER OF FOOD OPTIMISING

In the next sections you will be amazed and thrilled to discover how you can:

- Base your meals on foods that fill you up so well, you can enjoy as much of them as you like (**Free Food**).
- Fill up on foods that speed your weight loss (**Speed Foods**).
- Be sure you are enjoying foods that boost vitamins and minerals, calcium and fibre (**Healthy Extras**).
- Enjoy foods that all diets typically ban (**Syns**).

The reason why Food Optimising is so effective and powerful is that it's based on SYNERGY (the magical process by which, when you put individual elements together, they produce results that are much more powerful than they would be on their own). Together, the balance of Free Food, Healthy Extras and Syns produces a synergy that allows Food Optimisers to eat to their appetite's content AND be confident that they are losing weight in a way that's bang in line with current thinking on nutrition.

And if that isn't magical enough, when they join a warm, friendly Slimming World group, members find there is an incredibly powerful synergy there too. They discover the sensational synergy between:

- **Food Optimising** – the revolutionary eating plan that changes lives.
- **IMAGE Therapy** – a unique system of motivation and support.
- **Body Magic** – the way that even dedicated couch potatoes can become active, get fitter and feel healthier – and enjoy it!

The next few short sections of this introduction go into a little more detail about how this synergy works in practice, and the sound nutrition sense behind it all that ensures that Slimming World members are eating healthily while achieving their weight-loss goals.

Don't worry if you're not so keen on the 'science bit' but just want to get on with cooking the irresistible recipes! The beauty of Food Optimising is that you don't need an in-depth knowledge of nutrition, or loads of spare time in which to analyse everything you put in your mouth: the principles of Food Optimising take care of all that for you.

We hope though that the more you find out about eating the Slimming World way, the more you'll want to explore. And with so many faddy and 'miracle' diets around, before embarking on a weight-loss campaign it's more important than ever to establish that the system you choose really does offer you the healthy, effective and realistic solution you're looking for.

As your introduction to lifelong healthy eating for the 21st century, *Free Foods* is light years ahead of those early cookery books. And we hope you'll enjoy discovering how Food Optimising and Slimming World are light years ahead in healthy weight management. Welcome to *Free Foods*, welcome to Food Optimising and welcome to Slimming World – the most slimmer-friendly way of losing weight and maintaining your healthy weight that you will find anywhere.

FREE TO EAT

Free Food is at the heart of Food Optimising and is the key to its amazing success because it allows slimmers to achieve what many people – especially the 'diet experts' – believe is impossible: to eat unlimited quantities of food, whenever they like, and still lose weight.

In fact, at this point you may be starting to feel a little sceptical yourself. After all, overeating is one of the main reasons why people put on weight, so how can encouraging slimmers to eat as much as they like ever hope to solve the problem? So let's be clear from the outset:

- **Food Optimising** – is based on sound science and mainstream nutrition thinking, not half-baked theories or fashionable obsessions.
- **Food Optimising** – is based on the scientific fact, agreed by all the experts, that losing weight is a question of altering your 'energy balance'.
- **This means** – taking in less energy (in the form of calories, or energy units) than you expend, so your body uses up surplus energy stored as fat.

This is why many traditional weight-loss diets are based on measuring: measuring the number of calories in your food, measuring exactly how much you take in, in the form of calories or some other unit representing calories, and measuring how many calories you are burning down at the gym. Furthermore, conventional weight-loss systems require you to focus on the number of calories you are cutting down on in the form of food.

Simultaneously, such weight-loss systems also ask you to focus on how much you are increasing your output of calories in the form of exercise. And while this is a very sound scientific theory, what happens, all too often, when it is oversimplified and put into practice without any consideration of how people actually feel and behave?

CALORIE COUNTING

On a restrictive, calorie-counting diet, sooner or later the body and mind begin to rebel: the body feels deprived of satisfying meals and begins to crave the comfort of food, while the mind starts to obsess on the foods it is being denied and feelings of deprivation. Measuring and weighing everything we eat or drink becomes first a bore, and then a hated chore. Eventually many slimmers reach the point where they can't even bear to hear the word 'calorie'.

This is not the way to get slim or stay slim. What's more, scientists also agree that the weight-loss process is most effective when it happens gradually. A sudden, sharp reduction in calorie intake (as in a 'crash diet') results in the loss of more lean body tissue (such as muscle) from the body as well as body fat. Loss of lean tissue has unfavourable effects on our metabolic rate: the more we lose, the more our metabolic rate will fall.

As thousands of slimmers discover every week to their delight, Food Optimising is nothing at all like this!

- **On the contrary**, the revolutionary concept of Free Foods, which you can eat without restriction, whenever and wherever you need to eat, does away with the tyranny of calorie counting and the risks of crash dieting in one single stroke of genius.
- **What's more, with Food Optimising** Free Foods aren't just the watery and bland 'diet foods' you might expect, such as carrot sticks and cottage cheese!
- **The fantastic range of Free Foods** available to Food Optimisers includes pasta, rice, potatoes, lean meat, fish, poultry, and all the fresh fruit and vegetables you can eat – all without having to weigh, measure or count a single spoonful.

The starriest of celebrity chefs would love to have a list of Food Optimising Free Foods in his or her larder! Think of the wonderful, tasty, filling meals you can make with all those foods to choose from: a huge plate of pasta with a rich roast vegetable sauce; a spicy potato and spinach curry with a mountain of fluffy rice; or a big juicy fillet steak, cooked to your liking, with a jacket potato and a chunky salad. How about a big Spanish omelette, some tomato and monkfish kebabs, a roast dinner with plenty of lean meat and vegetables, or a full English cooked breakfast?

All of these meals – and so many more besides, as you'll find in this book – can be eaten freely when you are following Food Optimising. All you have to decide is whether to have a Green or an Original day (there's more about this on page 21).

By now you'll have realised why we're so sure that Food Optimising is nothing like those restrictive diets that depend on you counting and measuring every bite! But how do Free Foods achieve that shift in energy balance that scientists agree is essential for successful weight loss?

FREE FOOD SYNERGY

The answer lies in a remarkable synergy of the kind referred to in the first chapter: that between Slimming World's understanding of the emotional and psychological needs of slimmers, and the latest, up-to-the-minute scientific thinking on the relationship between appetite, overeating and dieting.

- **By basing** your daily eating on Free Foods when you are Food Optimising, you will be satisfying your appetite on foods that fill you up most effectively and keep you feeling fuller for longer.
- **This means** – you will automatically be limiting your overall calorie intake – without counting a single calorie!
- **You will also** – feel less need for high fat, high sugar snacks that pile on the calories, and the pounds, without providing any nutritional benefit.

Our appetite is regulated by many signals to the brain that arise as we digest our food, from chewing right through to absorption of the nutrients we've consumed. Food Optimising incorporates the latest scientific understanding of the foods that trigger the signal to stop eating when our body doesn't need any more (satiation) and the signal that prevents us from wanting to eat again until we need more energy (satiety). Research sponsored by Slimming World shows that of the major food groups, foods rich in protein (e.g. lean meat and fish) or carbohydrate (pasta and potatoes) are most effective in filling us up and keeping us feeling fuller for longer, while fat trails a long way behind. And these foods, which are the most important in triggering these signals of satiation and satiety, form the basis of Slimming World's revolutionary Free Foods list.

Many foods that are rich in carbohydrates or proteins also have another bonus for slimmers: they are relatively low in energy density, which means that weight for weight, they are low in calories. A highly energy-dense food, such as chocolate, for example, packs a large number of calories into a small volume. A low energy-dense food, such as a jacket potato, has far fewer calories, weight for weight. This means that low energy-dense foods take time to eat; they are bulky, which makes it harder to overeat on them. Highly energy-dense foods – typically those that have a lot of fat, oil or sugar – can be eaten quickly, so that it's easy to consume a lot of calories in a short time without even noticing. Free Foods are the key to your slimming success because they're just packed full of power. For an idea of just how powerful Free Foods are, see the box at the top of the page overleaf.

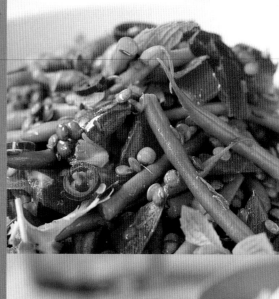

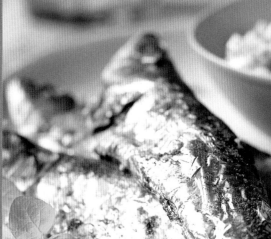

- **Filling power**: Free Foods are relatively low in energy density and are bulky too, so they fill you up and make it more difficult to consume a lot of calories.
- **Satisfying power**: Free Foods keep you feeling fuller for longer than other foods, so you don't feel the need to eat until you require more energy.
- **Slimming power**: Free Foods help you to make healthier food choices automatically, limiting your calorie intake and ensuring you lose weight – without counting a single calorie.
- **Liberating power**: Free Foods unlock the door to a feeling of freedom and relaxation around food that magically lightens the burden of slimming.
- **Appetite-reducing power**: Free Foods reduce your appetite naturally and healthily with the combined synergistic effect of all these physical and psychological weight-loss boosters.

BEING EMPOWERED

The second part of the answer to the apparent mystery of how Food Optimising can encourage slimmers to eat as much Free Food as they like, whenever they like, lies in Slimming World's passionate desire for slimmers to feel free, relaxed and in control around food. Far too many people with a weight problem live in fear: fear of 'eating too much', fear of 'forbidden foods', fear of being 'bad' for being overweight and fear of being judged and discounted. Then, if and when they try to tackle their problem with a diet, a whole new set of fears takes over: fear of failure, fear of being hungry, fear of being 'told off' for failing, and fear of foods they begin to believe are 'bad'.

The result, all too often, is a demoralising cycle of being 'on a diet' and 'off the diet' again, in which every single pound that you have struggled so hard to lose gradually creeps back on, and probably with a few more besides.

Slimming World's approach is designed to banish all these fears and the self-defeating behaviour they produce. Food Optimising replaces the need for cast-iron willpower with liberating 'choice power'. Our experience over many years has shown us that, given unrestricted access to a wide range of foods, slimmers do not go 'overboard'. That said, when they first join Slimming World, some of our members are feeling as doubtful as you might be now, and set out to 'prove us wrong' by eating as much Free Food as possible in their first week! Invariably, they are delighted to eat their words, as it were, when they discover they have had a better weight loss than they've ever had on a strict diet.

The liberating effect of realising that they have 'choice power' is strengthened by the positive, supportive energy members experience in their warm, friendly Slimming World group. Here they quickly find they are treated as capable, competent adults rather than naughty children who must be lectured or told off for their eating habits.

- **Freed from the fear of hunger** – their need to overeat disappears.
- **Freed from the fear of being judged, criticised or humiliated** – they find they begin to make healthy choices naturally and confidently.
- **Behaviour around food** becomes more rational.
- **Decisions** become real, not enforced.
- **Motivation** soars as fantastic results begin straightaway and continue weekly.

Free Food unlocks the door to freedom, choice and variety – heaven for slimmers who associate weight-loss regimes with restrictions, rules and monotony! And as we will see in the next sections, there are even more powerful synergies at work to ensure that Food Optimising is the most generous, most flexible, most satisfying and most slimmer-friendly way of losing weight and maintaining your healthy weight you can find.

SPEED IT UP!

No food can be said to be 'fattening' or 'slimming' on its own, as it's your overall diet that determines whether you lose weight, gain weight or stay the same. That said, some foods can be especially helpful to slimmers because they are even lower in energy density than other foods in the same group. Weight for weight, they have fewer calories than similar foods – so they're wonderfully filling and beautifully slimming.

At Slimming World, we've identified these super-slimmer-friendly foods and named them Speed Foods. They include a wide range of Free Foods, including favourites like chicken and fish, and many fruits and vegetables, and some Healthy Extra choices are also Speed Foods. Super Speed Foods are extra-low in calories, weight for weight, and they are all Free Foods.

Many Slimming World members find that their weight loss rolls along very well without having to choose Speed Foods specifically. But basing more meals on Speed Foods can be useful if you find your weight loss is a bit slower than you'd like, or if your lifestyle has changed – for example because you've become less active.

In their Slimming World group, members learn about the full range of Speed Foods and how to use them in everyday eating. Eating more Speed Foods is a way that Food Optimisers can give their weight loss a boost without cutting down on Syns – yet another way that Slimming World achieves the seemingly impossible for slimmers.

FREE TO CHOOSE

WITH FOOD OPTIMISING, you can forget diet plans that tell you to put your food on smaller plates to make the portions look bigger. We have already seen how Free Food allows you to make healthier food choices naturally, ensuring you can lose weight while piling even the biggest plate – and going back for seconds if you like.

Now it's time to discover the other clever ways in which Food Optimising helps to make your 'choice power' even more effective.

Each day, we ask you to choose between two styles of menu – Green or Original. It sounds easy – but it can be tricky deciding which you prefer, as they're both super-healthy and super-delicious. Most Food Optimisers base their choice on what they're doing and what they fancy eating that day.

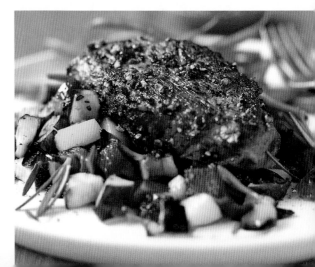

THE GREEN CHOICE

On these days you can eat lots of filling, healthy carbohydrates, plus generous servings of protein for a balanced diet, low in fat.

The Green choice is for days when you feel like filling up on comforting pasta, jacket potatoes, vegetable curries and chillies. Enjoy unlimited pasta, rice, potatoes, baked beans, pulses and grains, plus vegetables, fresh fruit, very low-fat natural yogurt and fromage frais.

A typical Green day meal could include a pile of pasta with spicy tomato sauce, topped with a measured serving of grilled chicken plus a large salad, followed with a big bowl of fresh pineapple and very low-fat fromage frais.

THE ORIGINAL CHOICE

The Original choice incorporates plenty of lean, satisfying protein, plus energising carbohydrates for a balanced diet, low in fat.

Go Original when you feel like treating yourself to an all-day egg and bacon breakfast, roast beef, fresh fish or seafood. Enjoy unlimited lean beef, lamb, pork (including bacon), chicken, turkey, fish and seafood, plus fresh fruit and most vegetables, very low-fat natural yogurt and fromage frais.

A typical Original day meal might be a juicy lean steak, as big as you like, with a measured portion of new potatoes in their skins and a big heap of broccoli, carrots and cauliflower. For pudding, treat yourself to fresh strawberries smothered in creamy, very low-fat natural yogurt.

MAKE YOUR CHOICE

Which choice is better? Neither – they're both great! Some Food Optimisers prefer to stick to Green days, some to Original days, and many opt for the Gold choice – alternating Green and Original days for maximum variety and superb results.

As you'll see from our suggestions for Green and Original day meals, Food Optimising is nothing like food combining, where protein-rich and carbohydrate-rich foods are not allowed to be eaten together in the same meal. Instead, Food Optimising is all about a healthy balance – filling up on the satisfying foods that you feel like eating that day, balanced with smaller portions of other foods to make everyday, family meals with added Food Optimising magic! Some foods are Free on both the Green and the Original choice, to provide even greater flexibility. These include:

- Some non-meat proteins, such as **Quorn** and **tofu**.
- **Eggs**, which are high in protein.
- **Fruit** and **green vegetables**, which are rich in complex carbohydrates.
- Very low-fat **natural yogurt**, **fromage frais** and **cottage cheese**.

You can add these freely to meals whenever you like as well as filling up on the foods that are Free on the choice you have chosen for that day.

FLEXIBILITY IS ALL

At Slimming World we understand that to be successful and effective, a healthy-eating plan has to fit into your lifestyle, not the other way round. Food Optimising frees you from so many restrictions that slimmers often feel are an inevitable part of the misery of 'dieting'. So, with Food Optimising you can:

- **Accept invitations** to restaurants and parties, confident that you will be able to enjoy the food along with everyone else.
- **Cook meals** the whole family will enjoy instead of having to eat separate 'slimming' meals.
- **Enjoy traditional favourites**, such as fish and chips or eggs on toast, without having to make faddy compromises or splash out on expensive ingredients.

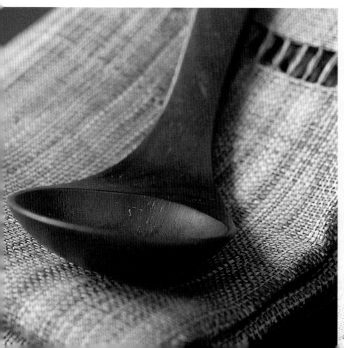
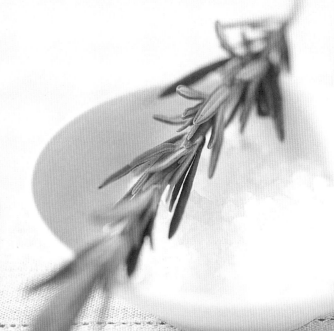

■ **Be confident** that you are following a healthy-eating plan, based on the latest in mainstream nutrition thinking, without having to be an expert on nutrition or scrutinising every food label.

Being able to mix and match your meals according to what you like eating and what you have planned for each day is wonderfully flexible and freeing, especially if you are used to weight-loss plans that dictate what you should eat at each meal, every day. Food Optimisers find that instead of being given a diet sheet, they are encouraged to plan their own daily and weekly menus from huge lists of ordinary, everyday, tasty foods.

Slimming World members are thrilled to discover that they are the ones in charge of what they eat – and that learning to manage their wide range of choices is not only easy, but fun! In this way, taking control of food choices soon becomes a habit, and soon after that, becomes second nature: a way of eating that can be maintained for life to ensure that weight problems become a thing of the past – forever.

FREE TO EXPLORE

W E HAVE ALREADY seen the powerful synergy between the sound nutrition principles of Food Optimising and the advanced behavioural science that underpins our Slimming World groups. And amazing though that is, there are many more synergies within Food Optimising that make it a truly revolutionary way of eating for managing your weight. To explore those synergies to the full, all you have to do is take three easy steps:

STEP 1: FILL UP ON FREE FOODS

Having decided whether you are going to have a Green or Original day, the first step to Food Optimising is to plan exactly which Free Foods you are going to satisfy your appetite with that day. On each choice there is a huge range of Free Foods to enjoy: we have given you some examples of Free Foods for both Green and Original days on pages 44–5.

Because Free Foods are so perfect for slimmers – tasty, versatile, filling and relatively low in energy density – you might think that you could eat well and lose weight just by sticking to Free Foods – and you'd be right. You'll be thrilled at just how particularly easy it is to put together satisfying, slimming meals without having to weigh, measure or count a single ingredient. But for maximum health benefits and variety, we at Slimming World then ask you to eat some more!

FIBRE, FRUIT AND FIVE A DAY

Eating plenty of fibre is important for our general health and it's especially useful for slimmers. Fibre-rich foods tend to be both bulky and relatively low in calories, so they're an efficient way to fill up when you're aiming to reduce your overall energy intake. Our national diet tends to be low in fibre, which increases our risk of developing various health problems, from constipation to more serious illnesses of the digestive system and even heart disease (as some forms of dietary fibre help to lower cholesterol).

Fruit and vegetables are fantastic for slimmers as they are high in fibre, packed with health-boosting vitamins and minerals, and relatively low in calories – which is why they're Free Food at Slimming World. Research shows

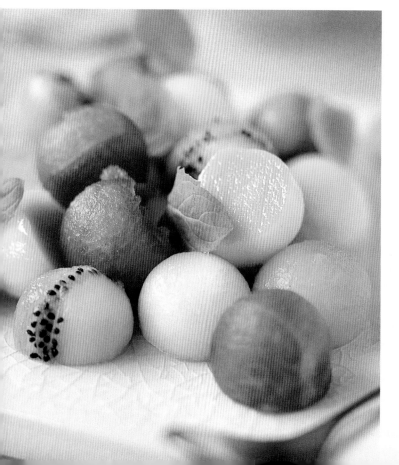

- When eating foods **high in fibre**, ensure you drink plenty of water to help digest it.
- On **Green** days, Free Foods high in fibre include: baked beans, chickpeas, lentils, peas, Quorn, red kidney beans and soya beans.
- On **Original** days, high-fibre Free Foods include artichokes, broccoli, Brussels sprouts, French beans, Quorn and runner beans.

that eating whole fruits and vegetables is better from a nutritional point of view than juices or purées, which is why these have a Syn value instead of being Free Food.

The Department of Health recommends that we eat five portions of fruit and vegetables every day for good health. We say have at least that! Potatoes don't count towards your 'five a day', but as they are filling, a good source of fibre and rich in vitamin C, you can enjoy them as Free Foods on Green days.

For optimum health, think about 'eating a rainbow' when it comes to choosing your fruit and vegetables. A huge range of vitamins, minerals and disease-fighting compounds is included in red, orange, yellow, dark green and purple produce. But all fruit and vegetables are beneficial to your health and your weight loss so don't worry if you don't like sprouts or strawberries – fill up on your favourites instead!

You can also add to the fibre content of food by choosing wholemeal bread and pasta, high-fibre breakfast cereals and soups, and by adding fibre-rich foods like beans or pulses to stews and bakes.

If your diet is currently low in fibre, your system may need a bit of help to process lots more fibre-rich food when you start Food Optimising. With this in mind, we suggest increasing your fibre intake slowly and it's always important to drink plenty of water, which is essential for good health and especially so for good digestion.

STEP 2: A QUESTION OF BALANCE

In addition to all the Free Foods, every day we ask you to choose three or four measured portions of Healthy Extras. Nutritionists agree that a healthy, balanced diet includes a daily intake of foods rich in fibre and calcium, vitamins and other minerals. Calcium especially is vital for good health; it's essential for strong bones and teeth, and helps nerves, muscle and blood to function properly. It may also help lower high blood pressure and protect against certain cancers. According to the latest research, calcium may play an important role in helping the body to reduce body fat, by altering the way in which fat cells function.

Healthy Extra choices include milk and cheese for calcium, and wholemeal bread, high-fibre breakfast cereals and soups for dietary fibre. On Green days, the Healthy Extras list includes lean meat, fish and poultry. On Original days, you could also choose potatoes, wholemeal pasta and pulses. In the Free Foods selections on pages 218–19, we include ideas for some Healthy Extras.

STEP 3: ENJOY A LITTLE SYNERGY!

After Free Foods and Healthy Extras, Syns are the third element that make Food Optimising the most effective weight-loss plan ever. Syns are the way that Food Optimising gives you a marvellous safety net, so that you can enjoy all the freewheeling you need to liberate yourself from hunger and deprivation, with just enough structure and control to ensure a motivating weight loss week after week.

Syns are also the way you can enjoy the foods that most diets ban – and without a shred of guilt! All foods that aren't Free on the day you've chosen have a Syn value. Counting the Syns you use each day helps you balance your diet for optimum weight loss, and maximum enjoyment.

As we've already seen, foods that are low in energy density are the most helpful for slimmers, which is why these foods are Free at Slimming World. Eating lots of foods that are high in energy density, such as fats and oils, sugar, alcohol – and processed foods that contain these ingredients – can sabotage any slimming campaign.

That's why we recommend that Food Optimisers limit the amount of highly energy-dense foods they are eating by allowing themselves an agreed number of Syns each day. No one will tell you how many Syns to have each day; it's up to you. For most people, a level of around 10–15 Syns each day is about right to keep the pounds melting away.

We don't tell you how to use your Syns either. Some people like to spend theirs on little extras like gravy, mayonnaise or pickles, to make meals even more delicious. Others prefer to have a glass or two of red wine, or a chocolate bar or a packet of crisps – and are thrilled they can enjoy treats like these every single day and still lose weight. For a list of the foods most often taken as Syns, see page 220.

SYNS: SAFETY NETS AND SAFETY VALVES

Even if you're losing weight happily by choosing 10 or 15 Syns a day, there will always be occasions when that's just too tight for comfort. An invitation to a wedding or a special party, a weekend away, even a terrible day at work – with many weight-loss systems, events like these can spell disaster. Unable to stick to the rules, slimmers throw caution to the winds and then agonise with guilt that they have 'blown it' completely. A 'bad' day turns into a 'bad' week, and suddenly there they are – a 'bad' person who's failed again.

At Slimming World we understand only too well that everyone needs a

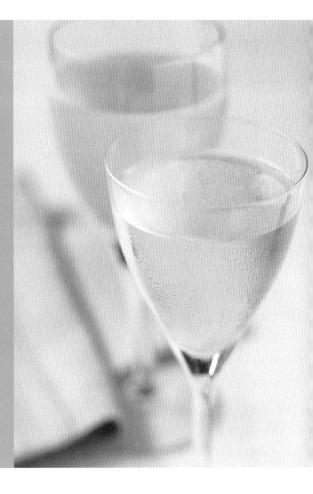

- **Flexible Syns** are another amazing aspect of Food Optimising: it seems impossible that you can go over your daily Syn allowance (and sometimes way, way over) and still lose weight. Yet it works.
- When you opt for flexible Syns we ask you to **stay aware**, and to **stay counting** – up to a total that you have agreed with yourself in advance.
- Suppose you are having that bad day at work and you decide you need a **special treat** to see you through until home-time. At lunch, you agree with yourself to have 20 Syns; you enjoy them, and keep counting. For the rest of the day and on the next day, you return to your **usual Syn allowance** – without trying to 'make up' for your lunchtime treat.
- You've stayed **aware** and **in control**. There is no need to feel you've 'failed', undone all your good work or that you will never be able to achieve your goal.

safety valve from time to time. Research evidence shows that being flexible when losing weight is the key to long-term success. So that's where 'flexible Syns' come in.

The secret of flexible Syns' success is based on Slimming World's understanding that if 20, 50 or even 100 Syns sounds like an awful lot, it's certainly fewer than if you'd stopped counting altogether, and less damaging than if you'd convinced yourself there was no point in trying again.

Together with Free Food and Healthy Extras, Syns and flexible Syns are the way that Food Optimising becomes truly enjoyable, completely versatile and easy to adopt as a way of eating healthily for life.

It's important to remember, though, that you don't have to focus on Syns to lose weight successfully. Free Food is the way that you satisfy your appetite, even on the hungriest days, and Free Food is how you learn to lose weight fast and keep it off for good. Then enjoy your Syns – they're the icing on the cake!

FREE TO GO

F ROM THE OUTSET we've established that Food Optimising is the complete opposite of crash dieting, which severely restricts your energy intake with the result that weight lost can include lean body tissue as well as fat – damaging for your metabolism and general health. Crash dieting just isn't possible when you're following the most generous weight-loss plan ever: Slimming World members generally enjoy 1500–1800 calories a day.

That said, many Slimming World members are delighted to report big weight losses in their first week of Food Optimising, and some go on to lose weight at a consistently fast rate. So what is a healthy rate of weight loss and what might you expect when you begin Food Optimising?

- Generally, we encourage a **healthy rate of weight loss**, averaging 500g–1kg (1–2lb) a week. This is an achievable goal for most people.
- Everyone is different and people lose weight at different rates influenced by a number of factors such as **genetics**, how much **weight** they have to lose, and how **active** they are.
- When people have quite a lot of weight to lose, it's not unusual to see **initial losses** of 3–4kg (7–10lb) in the first week and **more than** 500g–1kg (1–2lb) in the following few weeks, which is partly due to the loss of water.
- For most of our members, weight loss **settles** to 500g–1kg (1–2lb) per week.

Top medical advisors have confirmed to us that if people are Food Optimising properly, a rapid weight loss isn't a problem. As long as slimmers are eating plenty of food, having a balanced diet and exercising to help maintain lean muscle tissue, a weight loss of more than 500g–1kg (1–2lb) a week over several weeks or even months can still be perfectly healthy.

But as you'll find every step of the way at Slimming World, you're the one who's in control. We don't tell you how much weight you 'should' be losing, or dictate to you the weight you 'should' be aiming for. Where you want to go, and how fast or slowly you want to get there, is up to you. Some of our members take 'route one' straight to the target they've chosen, others take a more leisurely path with a few twists and turns along the way. That's fine by us; if you're happy, we're happy.

There is one weight-loss target we like everyone to be aware of, though, and that's when you've lost 10 per cent of your starting weight – for example, if you've slimmed from 20st to 18st. This is a reason to celebrate because medical evidence suggests that if you are very overweight, losing just 10 per cent of your starting weight brings substantial health benefits if you then maintain that loss for ten weeks or more. Losing 10 per cent of your body weight is an achievement to be proud of and we celebrate this at Slimming World by making you a member of our 'Club 10' scheme, with a further reward if you maintain your loss or go on to lose more in the next ten weeks (as many, many Club 10 members do).

GET GOING FOR SUCCESS!

All our experience at Slimming World tells us that having a good weight loss in your first week of Food Optimising is a marvellous motivator and a big step on the journey to success.

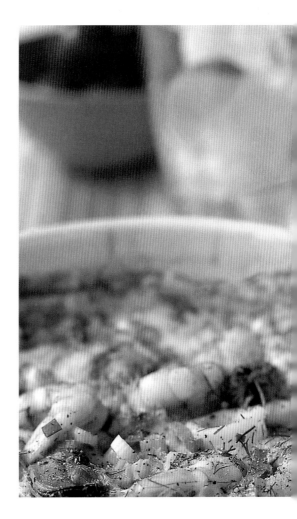

- **Work out** what you would love to eat at each meal over the next week, giving priority to Free Foods, then Healthy Extras, then Syns.
- **Plan your meals**, taking into account the demands on your time during the week ahead.
- Aim to **vary your choices** through the week and to cook meals the whole family will enjoy; there's no need to make separate meals just for yourself.
- Aim to **prepare ahead** as far as you can – take half an hour the night before to prepare the next day's meal, and make the most of slow cookers and automatic oven settings to make cooking **more convenient**.
- **Make a list** before you go food shopping and stick to it; but make sure you include the treats you plan to spend your Syns on so you don't feel deprived.
- **Test out Free Foods** to the limit and enjoy, relish and savour every mouthful you eat. Don't believe friends and family who say you can't eat all that and slim. They're wrong! You can!

FREE YOUR SPIRIT

Most of us who struggle with our weight would love more than just a slim body: we'd love a fit, healthy, active body too, with the fabulous light feeling that comes from being free to move around with lots of energy.

Becoming fitter and more active isn't just important for our health and wellbeing; the level of activity we do is the other element of the 'energy equation' that determines whether we lose or gain weight or stay the same. In the opinion of many medical experts, increasing the amount of energy we expend, while also reducing the amount of energy we consume as food, is the key to lasting weight loss. Regular exercise also brings many other benefits, both physical and psychological, ranging from a body that burns fat faster to a healthier immune system, higher self-esteem and less stress and anxiety.

As you would expect from the organisation that developed Food Optimising, Slimming World has taken its own unique and original approach to encouraging members to become active. And as you would also expect, our approach involves another powerful synergy, this time between Food Optimising and the right kind of moderate activity. We call it Body Magic.

The latest scientific evidence suggests that we don't have to go flat-out with intensive activity in order to reap the health benefits of getting fitter. Moderate, regular activity, such as walking briskly for 30 minutes several times a week, can be just as effective in helping us feel better, have more energy, and reduce some of the health risks faced by people who have very inactive lifestyles.

With more than 35 years' experience of helping slimmers make positive changes in their lives, Slimming World understands that developing the habit of exercise requires just as much support as developing healthy eating habits. We also recognise that everyone is at their own unique starting point when it comes to activity; some people are sporty and love to exercise, while others would find it a struggle to walk to the end of their street. Many members feel that they should be 'doing something' about exercise, but may have bad memories of school sports or simply find it difficult to make being active a priority.

DEVELOPING YOUR OWN REGIME

So instead of focusing on individual types of exercise or setting unattainable targets, Body Magic is an initiative that recognises and celebrates members' progress in developing an activity routine, measured in terms of time committed to exercise rather than physical performance.

This means that anyone can participate, since any step along the 'Activity Pathway' from a sedentary to a fully active lifestyle is supported and rewarded with praise and recognition within the group. For the member who spends her days in an armchair, walking to the corner shop is just as big an achievement as running a 5km race is for someone who is already a committed gym user.

Body Magic is fun! Each week, members are invited to decide how much more active they are going to be in the week ahead. They then note down all their activities in their personal FIT log (which stands for Frequency, Intensity, and Time spent). Over the weeks, members build up from the Bronze standard (45 minutes' exercise per week, spread over at least three days and maintained for four weeks) to the Gold standard (30 minutes of exercise, five days a week, maintained for eight weeks). And once a member feels that exercise has become an intrinsic part of their lifestyle – as natural and regular as cleaning their teeth – they achieve a Platinum award recognising lifelong Body Magic.

With the support of their Consultant, members explore why they may have been reluctant to exercise in the past and learn easy, enjoyable ways to boost their motivation such as 'foot out of the door' techniques – tricks such as putting your walking shoes by the TV remote, with a note reminding you not to switch on until you've stepped out!

Body Magic and Food Optimising have a magical synergy because they complement each other perfectly; one of the great benefits of exercise is that it boosts our mood and our self-esteem, so it is easier to feel calm, in control and in the right frame of mind to make healthy-eating choices. And the more

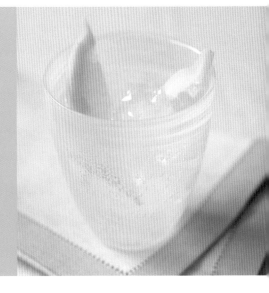

- With **Body Magic**, no one activity is recommended as being better than another.
- Members are encouraged to build **movement** and **activity** into everyday life wherever and whenever they can.
- Get off the **bus** a stop earlier and walk, use the **stairs** instead of the escalator, or **walk** the children to school and back instead of driving.
- The **positive**, inspiring atmosphere of a Slimming World group is the **ideal environment** for members to overcome the motivational barriers to becoming more active.

effective Food Optimising is, the more energy members have and the more confident they feel about taking up sport, exercise, or just becoming more mobile. Together with IMAGE Therapy (of which more in the next section), Food Optimising and Body Magic help to reinforce members' sense of purpose, and this is what makes our groups so powerful.

FREE TO BE YOU

ALL THE EXPERTS agree that the rapid growth in the number of people becoming obese in the UK is the most important issue in public health. Obesity doesn't just limit people's lifestyles; it shortens lives. It increases our risk of developing illnesses such as diabetes, stroke, heart disease and certain cancers. In recognising the severity of the problem, the public health authorities are struggling to develop strategies to promote healthy weight management. Suggestions are made for drastic tactics, such as taxing high-fat foods or banning the advertising of snacks and sweets. Earnest academics call for the return of the 'Nanny state' and urge the Government to lay down the law to make us take more care of our weight and health.

The message sounds simple enough: eat more healthily and exercise more. Yet with over 35 years' experience of helping slimmers, Slimming World knows just how difficult it can be to make even a small lifestyle change, especially as the 21st century is a very unhelpful environment for slimmers. Our lives are more comfortable now than at any time in our evolutionary history. Far from having to hunt and forage for food over many miles as our Stone Age ancestors did, we only have to stretch out a hand for a processed, calorie-packed snack. At work, at home and at play, our lives are less energy-intensive and more sedentary than ever.

To decide to do things differently; to swim against the tide and consciously adopt new routines and habits that aren't easily deterred by setbacks and distractions, takes courage, determination and a positive outlook. It takes more than a strict talking-to from a 'Nanny' figure (Government-backed or otherwise) for people to feel they have the support, the encouragement and the unconditional approval they need to change their lives, permanently and for the better.

Nannies, of course, are for children, and the 'experts' who recommend a prescriptive, restrictive approach to weight management often give the impression that slimmers should be treated like children – as if they need to be told what to do to 'get on the straight and narrow'. The Slimming World approach could not be more different.

- We know our members are **adults**, not children.
- We appreciate our members for the **able**, **competent**, **warm**, **friendly** people they are – people who are more than capable of making their own decisions and achieving their goals.
- Within a group, our members are **valued**, **supported** and **respected**.

SLIMMING WORLD'S MUTUAL SUPPORT

The warm, positive atmosphere of a Slimming World group is no accident. It is born out of a deep understanding of what it's like to have a weight problem, and a philosophy that dieting alone is not the solution to long-term weight management. It is fostered by our Consultants, who have all been Slimming World members themselves and know how hard it can be to join a group and how vital it is to feel accepted and welcomed straight away. Many of our members are unhappy about themselves before they join us; their self-esteem is low and, based on what they've heard about slimming clubs, or on previous bad experiences, they fully expect to be made to feel worse.

Instead, they find plenty of praise and support, from the moment they first join the group and then on every single step of their weight-loss journey, and not just when things are going well but also when – especially when – things aren't going so well. When you know you've had a difficult week, it takes courage and commitment to go back to your group because it would be so much easier to stay away (and not come back the next week either). It's this courage and commitment that will get you to your chosen target and, at Slimming World, we know you'll need help and support. Your fellow members and Consultant understand this and applaud you for it.

IMAGE THERAPY

The other big surprise awaiting new members who have preconceived ideas about slimming clubs is that there is no lecture from a superior slim being! Instead, the whole group participates in a unique form of problem-sharing and problem-solving to which everyone is encouraged to contribute (although no one is singled out if they prefer to watch and listen). Our celebrated

IMAGE Therapy (Individual Motivation and Group Experience) is one of the most powerful support systems ever created, and of everything we do at Slimming World, it's probably the element we're proudest of. Through IMAGE Therapy, members are encouraged to:

- **Develop** their own insights into the psychological and practical barriers that get in the way of their weight-loss success.
- **Think through** their own techniques for overcoming them.
- **Share** the ups and downs of slimming so they learn, to their enormous relief, that there is virtually no problem or emotion that someone else hasn't already faced and overcome.

In this way, members experience an intoxicating mixture of inspiration and motivation that leaves them feeling cared for, worthwhile and valued.

EXERCISE YOUR CHOICE POWER

As we saw earlier, Food Optimising is all about replacing iron willpower with freeing, exhilarating choice power. In IMAGE Therapy, members learn how to use choice power for maximum effect in all areas of their lives. IMAGE Therapy puts the decision-making where it belongs – with the individual – and how empowering is that?

It starts with deciding the amount of weight you would like to lose. Your Personal Achievement Target (PAT) is just that: it's up to you to decide the point at which you would like to celebrate your success. Of course, if you feel, once you've got there, that you would like to set a new, lower personal target,

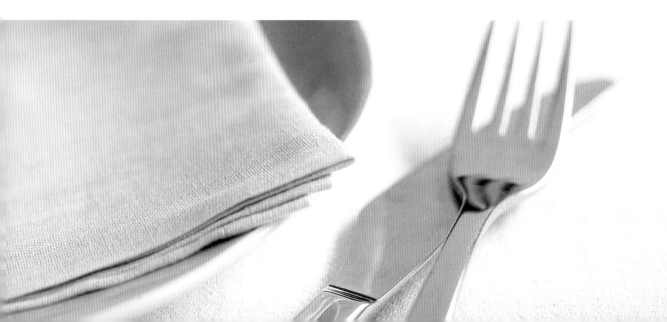

that's fine too. Setting your own weight-loss targets (which you don't have to share with the group) puts you totally in control of the process. And it removes at a stroke that terrible sense of failure if you decide you're happy just a few pounds short of a target that someone else thinks you should reach – no matter how much weight you've already lost and what your personal dreams are.

Setting your own target weight is a big decision, and at Slimming World members learn a lot about all the other daily decisions we make and their consequences. Just as there are no 'good' foods or 'bad' foods, there are no good or bad decisions at Slimming World – just choices that take you in different directions. Each week, members are asked to set themselves a weight-loss goal for the week ahead, and to think about the choices they might face.

For example, if your week includes a party, you might choose to abandon Food Optimising completely for the evening. Or you might choose to use flexible Syns, enjoy your evening and stay in control, or you might choose to offer to drive and keep to your usual Syns allowance for the day. Each of those choices will have a consequence for your weight-loss goal and none of them is the 'right' choice – the key is to be aware of the choices that will help you achieve your goal directly, and those that will take you on a more scenic route.

Just as Food Optimising empowers slimmers to make healthier food choices, IMAGE Therapy helps our members to make healthier life choices in an equally natural way. By finding that other people have faith in them, our members begin to exercise their 'choice muscles' and discover they are more capable, creative and assertive than they ever thought they could be. Losing weight may not transform our members' lives, but it gives them the unbeatable feeling that having succeeded once, they can achieve anything they desire – and quite frequently they go on to do just that!

In this introduction to our latest recipe collection, *Free Foods*, we can only give you a brief insight into the fantastic synergies that Slimming World has to offer to members. There is just one element missing that's needed to create the most powerful synergy of all – and that's you! If you join us at Slimming World, you will find out so much more about how to make Food Optimising and Body Magic part of your new lifestyle, and how to harness the power of IMAGE Therapy to make your weight loss dreams come true. You will also have the warmth and encouragement of your Consultant and fellow members to help you.

We hope you have many happy hours of cooking and eating the marvellous recipes in this book. We hope too that you will discover that *Free Foods* is more than a cookery book – even a modern, glossy, 21st-century cookery book! *Free Foods* is simply amazing; *Free Foods* is a recipe for life.

TAKE A WEEK or two to follow our tasty selection of mouth-watering menus and you'll be able to plan your shopping with confidence. You'll soon discover that not only does Food Optimising work, it's fabulously simple too!

These menus are designed to help you understand the variety of meals that are possible when you start Food Optimising. You're sure to have plenty of nourishing food that will keep you full and healthy – and help you to lose weight. In these menus we have included some of the recipes in this book. Please feel free to swap and change these for any of the other recipes if you'd prefer.

HERE'S HOW TO USE FOOD OPTIMISING MENUS MOST EFFECTIVELY:

1 Decide whether you wish to have a Green or Original day and stick to that choice all day. You can make every day a Green day or include some Original days too. Within the Green menus we have included meat-free choices suitable for vegetarians.

2 Pick one breakfast, one lunch and one dinner from your chosen set.

3 Choose around 10 to 15 Syns-worth of food from the Syns list on page 220. Some Food Optimisers find they lose weight best on 5 Syns, others on 20 Syns. On some days, you might find you perhaps need to use 30, if you are going out or celebrating. In general, we find 10 Syns a day is a good rule of thumb for effective weight loss.

4 Each day, choose twice from the following milk and cheese lists to boost your calcium intake, which is vital for a healthy diet.

Milk

- 350ml/12fl oz skimmed milk
- 250ml/8fl oz semi-skimmed milk
- 175ml/6fl oz whole milk
- 250ml/8fl oz calcium-enriched soya milk (sweetened or unsweetened)

Cheese

- 25g/1oz Cheddar
- 25g/1oz Edam
- 25g/1oz Gouda
- 40g/1½oz Mozzarella
- 40g/1½oz reduced fat Cheddar/Cheshire
- 3 triangles Original Dairylea
- 2 mini Babybel cheeses

Drink black tea, coffee (sweetened with artificial sweetener) and low-calorie drinks freely, and use fat-free French or vinaigrette-style salad dressings freely.

On the menus that are given on the following pages – divided into Green days and Original days – check out the foods that are marked in bold. These can be eaten freely without any weighing or measuring. Fill up on these foods when you feel peckish. You can also turn to our Free Food list on pages 218–19 and select other Free Foods to enjoy whenever you want, in whatever quantity you want.

Maximise your healthy eating by:

- Eating at least five portions of fresh fruit and vegetables every day.
- Trimming any visible fat off meat and removing any skin from poultry.
- Remembering the latest recommendations regarding intake of fluids, which is to aim for six to eight cups, mugs or glasses of any type of fluid per day (excluding alcohol).

Note for Slimming World members: Healthy Extra B choices are built into the menus.

When you have experienced the pleasure of Food Optimising on your plate you will want to make your own menus. You can do this with the complete Food Optimising system, available at Slimming World groups throughout the UK.

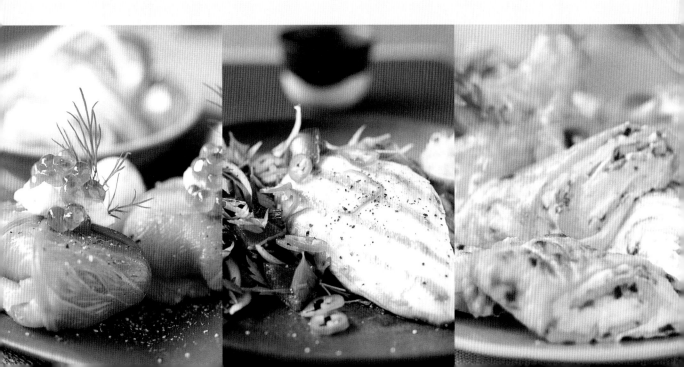

BREAKFASTS

1 Fresh **melon** wedges followed by 25g/1oz Shredded Wheat Honey Nut served with milk from the allowance and topped with heaps of fresh **strawberries**.

2 Two slices wholemeal bread, toasted and topped with oodles of **spaghetti hoops/baked beans** in tomato sauce, plus an **apple** and **banana**.

3 3 rashers grilled lean bacon, poached **egg**, grilled **tomatoes** and **mushrooms**, plus a **peach**.

4 Yogurt crunch made with **very low-fat natural yogurt**, 25g/1oz Jordans Special Muesli and sliced **kiwi**: layer the kiwi, muesli and yogurt right to the top of a tall glass finishing with a sprinkling of muesli and a slice of kiwi, followed by a **banana**.

5 A large fluffy **omelette** filled with grilled **mushrooms**, **tomatoes** and 25g/1oz grated Cheddar cheese and served with plenty of **baked beans** in tomato sauce, plus a **nectarine**.

6 Large bowl of fresh **orange** and **grapefruit** segments, sweetened with artificial sweetener if desired, followed by two Weetabix served with milk from the allowance and topped with lots of fresh **raspberries**.

7 Two slices wholemeal bread, toasted and topped with scrambled or poached **eggs**, followed by a bowl of fresh **strawberries** and **melon balls** topped with a **Müllerlight yogurt** (any variety).

8 25g/1oz Alpen or bran flakes topped with a pile of **blueberries** and served with milk from the allowance followed by heaps of sautéed sliced **potatoes** served with lots of grilled **mushrooms** and **baked beans** in tomato sauce.

9 **Quorn sausages**, grilled and served with lots of grilled **tomatoes**, **onion** wedges and poached or scrambled **eggs** and two slices of wholemeal toast, plus an **apple** and **peach**.

10 Fresh **grapefruit**, sweetened with artificial sweetener if desired, followed by 25g/1oz Shreddies topped with lots of sliced **banana** and served with milk from the allowance and a pot of **Marks & Spencer Count On Us Yogurt** (any variety).

LUNCHES

1 Basil and Tomato Pesto Pasta (see page 160) followed by 275g/10oz blackberries stewed and sweetened with artificial sweetener, if desired, and topped with plenty of **very low-fat natural yogurt.**

2 Large **jacket potato** filled with 25g/1oz grated Cheddar cheese and plenty of **baked beans** in tomato sauce served with a huge fresh **salad**. Plus an **apple** and **banana.**

3 Herbed Couscous Salad (see page 201) followed by 400g/14oz fruit cocktail canned in juice topped with lots of **very low-fat natural fromage frais.**

4 Cabbage and Carrot Stir-Fry (see page 146) served on a bed of **noodles**, followed by 275g/10oz apple and 275g/10oz rhubarb stewed and sweetened with artificial sweetener, if desired, and topped with a **Müllerlight vanilla yogurt.**

5 175g/6oz plaice fillet, grilled or poached and served with **Baby Roasted Potatoes with Fennel and Lemon Thyme** (see page 149) and a large mixed **salad**. Plus a large bowl of fresh **fruit** salad made with lots of chopped **melon, kiwi, strawberries** and **mango.**

6 Fruity Pasta Salad with Oranges and Grapes (see page 198) followed by 350g/12oz pears canned in juice and topped with a generous serving of **very low-fat natural yogurt.**

7 50g/2oz wholemeal crusty roll filled with lots of sliced **egg, tomato** and mixed **salad leaves**, followed by a large bowl of **strawberries** and **raspberries** layered with a pot of **Sainsbury's Be Good to Yourself yogurt** (any variety).

8 Baked Stuffed Peppers (see page 58) served with a large mixed **salad** and followed by 225g/8oz apple, baked and filled with 1 level tablespoon of mincemeat and topped with plenty of **very low-fat natural fromage frais.**

9 Sweetcorn and Coriander Soup (see page 52) plus a bowl of chopped fresh **pineapple** and **melon** topped with lots of **very low-fat natural yogurt** flavoured with **vanilla** and sprinkled with 2 level dessertspoons chopped mixed nuts.

10 100g/4oz skinless and boneless chicken breast, grilled and served with **Mixed Mushroom Noodle Stir-Fry** (see page 158) and a large **salad**, followed by an **orange** and lots of fresh **cherries** and/or **grapes.**

DINNERS

1 **Spinach and Sweet Potato Curry** (see page 142) served with heaps of steamed **Basmati rice**, followed by an **apple** and **satsuma**.

2 **Chunky Spaghetti Bolognese** (see page 164) followed by a huge selection of fresh **berries** topped with spoonfuls of **very low-fat natural fromage frais** flavoured with **vanilla**.

3 A large **omelette** filled with chopped **peppers**, **red onions** and **sweetcorn** and served with lots of baked **potato** wedges and loads of **salad**. Plus half a canteloupe **melon** piled high with **raspberries**.

4 **Cumin-Scented Chickpea Falafels** (see page 60) served with heaps of **couscous** and plenty of **roasted vegetables**. Plus lots of **strawberries** topped with a **Müllerlight yogurt** (any variety).

5 **Creamy Asparagus Carbonara** (see page 165), followed by a large bowl of chopped **apple**, **pear** and **grapes** topped with lots of **very low-fat natural yogurt**.

6 **Egg, Chip and Pepper Bake** (see page 178) served with a large mixed **salad** and followed by a tropical fresh **fruit** salad made with lots of chopped **mango**, **kiwi** and **papaya**.

7 **Glamorgan Sausages with Tomato Sauce** (see page 84) served with mountains of mashed **potatoes** and plenty of **peas**, **carrots** and **sweetcorn**. Plus lots of sliced **banana** topped with a **Müllerlight toffee yogurt** and sprinkled with **cinnamon**.

8 Vegetable stir-fry: **broccoli** and **cauliflower** florets, chopped **carrots**, mixed **peppers**, **spring onions**, button **mushrooms**, **beansprouts** and **water chestnuts** stir-fried with **garlic**, **herbs** and **soy sauce** served on a generous bed of **noodles**, plus an **apple**.

9 **Couscous with Stewed Vegetables** (see page 172) followed by a large bowl of **raspberries** topped with **very low-fat natural fromage frais** sweetened with artificial sweetener if desired.

10 Large **jacket potato** topped with a can of **mixed beans** in chilli sauce and served with a generous mixed **salad**, plus a **peach** and lots of fresh **cherries** and/or **grapes**.

BREAKFASTS

1 Fresh **grapefruit**, sweetened with artificial sweetener if desired, plus lots of lean grilled **gammon**, grilled **tomatoes** and **mushrooms**, poached **egg** and served with two slices of wholemeal bread, toasted.

2 **Melon** boat filled with lots of fresh **summer fruits**, topped with **very low-fat natural yogurt** and sprinkled with 25g/1oz Shredded Wheat Fruitful.

3 250g/9oz raspberries stewed with artificial sweetener to taste, topped with a **Müllerlight country berries yogurt**, followed by plenty of grilled **kippers**, **tomatoes** and **onion** wedges.

4 Two Weetabix served with milk from the allowance followed by a large fluffy **omelette** filled with lots of lean **ham** and **mushrooms**.

5 Two slices wholemeal bread, toasted and topped with scrambled **egg** mixed with chopped smoked **salmon** and **chives** and served with grilled **tomatoes**, followed by a few **plums**.

6 A large bowl of fresh **orange** and **grapefruit** segments, followed by 40g/1½oz Kellogg's All Bran Apricot Bites served with milk from the allowance and topped with lots of sliced **banana**.

7 Lots of lean grilled **bacon**, **mushrooms**, poached **egg** and served with 150g/5oz baked beans in tomato sauce, followed by a bowl of chopped **kiwi** and **strawberries** smothered in **Müllerlight yogurt** (any variety).

8 50g/2oz wholemeal crusty roll filled with lots of grilled **mackerel** fillets topped with slices of fresh **tomato**, followed by a selection of **melon** wedges.

9 Banana split: **banana** sliced lengthways, sprinkled with 40g/1½oz Kellogg's All Bran Original and topped with oodles of **very low-fat natural yogurt** flavoured with **cinnamon**.

10 Two slices of wholemeal bread, toasted and topped with plum **tomatoes** with a dash of Worcestershire sauce followed by a **peach** and lots of **cherries** and/or **grapes**.

LUNCHES

1 Fresh **tuna** or **swordfish** steak baked in the oven with **coriander** and **lime juice** served with a large mixed **salad** and 200g/7oz new potatoes boiled in their skins, followed by a bunch of **grapes**.

2 Asparagus and Ham Open Egg White Omelette (see page 192) followed by 225g/8oz apple baked and 100g/4oz blackberries, stewed and topped with lots of **very low-fat natural yogurt** flavoured with **vanilla**.

3 All-Day Breakfast Salad (see page 209) served with a 50g/2oz wholemeal crusty roll, followed by a bowl of **strawberries** and chopped **melon**.

4 Parchment Fish Parcels (see page 130) served with a large mixed **salad** and a 225g/8oz jacket potato (raw weight) followed by lots of **apple** and **orange** segments topped with **very low-fat natural fromage frais**.

5 Stuffed Chicken and Courgette 'Sandwich' (see page 81) followed by 225g/8oz apple, baked and topped with 1 level tablespoon mincemeat smothered in **Müllerlight yogurt** (any variety).

6 Lean fillet **steak**, tossed in black **peppercorns**, grilled and served with 200g/7oz new potatoes in their skins, and lots of **baby whole sweetcorn**, **sugar snap peas** and **asparagus**. Plus a large fresh **fruit** salad: chopped **mango**, **peach** and **pineapple**.

7 Stuffed Tomato Salad (see page 78) served with two slices of wholemeal bread, followed by **melon** wedges sprinkled with fresh **raspberries**.

8 Spicy Pork Burgers (see page 86) served with a large mixed **salad**, followed by 200g/7oz apple and 225g/8oz blackcurrants stewed and layered with oodles of **very low-fat natural fromage frais**.

9 Seafood and Dill Omelette (see page 112) served with a big **salad** and 225g/8oz jacket potato (raw weight), followed by a **banana** and **pear**.

10 Roasted Yellow Pepper Soup (see page 50) served with a 50g/2oz wholemeal crusty roll, plus a bowl of chopped **mango**, **kiwi** and **papaya** topped with lashings of **very low-fat natural yogurt**.

DINNERS

1 **Italian-Style Stuffed Peaches** (see page 56) followed by a **chicken** breast, grilled or baked and served with loads of **red cabbage**, thin **green beans** and **butternut squash**.

2 **Comfort Food Fish Pie** (see page 115) followed by a large bowl of **raspberries**, **blackberries** and **blueberries** topped with **very low-fat natural fromage frais**.

3 **Melon** boat filled with **strawberries** followed by **Mustard and Garlic Roasted Leg of Lamb** (see page 98) served with lots of **asparagus**, **carrots** and **baby whole sweetcorn**.

4 **Spicy Beef and Vegetable Stew** (see page 108) followed by lots of fresh **mango** and sliced **grapes** topped with **very low-fat natural yogurt**.

5 Lean **gammon** steak, grilled, topped with fresh **pineapple** slices and served with a plateful of **salad leaves**, **cherry tomatoes**, **cucumber**, **spring onions** and grated **carrot**. Plus a **peach** or **nectarine**.

6 **Crusted Fillet Steak with Roast Vegetable Salsa** (see page 106) followed by **Minted Tropical Fruit Salad** (see page 206).

7 Slices of **honeydew melon** followed by **Grilled Tandoori Duck** (see page 97). Plus a bowl of **very low-fat natural yogurt** mixed with lots of sliced **banana** and **vanilla**.

8 Large **salmon** steak, sprinkled with **lemon juice** and chopped **parsley**, grilled or baked and served with heaps of **mangetout**, **baby carrots** and **baby whole sweetcorn**. Plus a large bowl of chopped **pineapple**, **kiwi**, **melon** and **strawberries**.

9 **Bangers and Mash** (see page 85) served with heaps of **cabbage**, **carrots** and **broccoli** followed by a **peach** and a few **plums**.

10 A bowl of fresh **orange** and **grapefruit** segments topped with **raspberries** followed by a lean boneless **pork** steak, grilled or baked, served with lots of oven roasted **vegetables**: chunks of **red**, **yellow** and **green pepper**, **red onion** wedges, **tomato** halves and a large **green salad**.

SYN-FREE STORECUPBOARD INGREDIENTS

All these storecupboard ingredients are **Free Foods** for both Original and Green days, unless otherwise stated.

CANS AND BOTTLES

Artificial **sweetener**

Baked beans in tomato sauce (Green days only)

Borlotti beans (Green days only)

Butter beans (Green days only)

Cannellini beans (Green days only)

Chickpeas (Green days only)

Fat-free dressings, French and vinaigrette style

Peppers

Pimento

Preserved **lemons**

Red kidney beans (Green days only)

Lean canned **ham** (Original days only)

Mackerel, in brine and in tomato sauce (Original days only)

Sardines, in brine and tomato sauce (Original days only)

Sweetcorn (Green days only)

Tomatoes, plum and chopped

Tuna, in brine and water (Original days only)

Water chestnuts

Capers and **caperberries**

Gherkins

STAPLES

Pearl barley (Green days only)

Bulgar wheat (Green days only)

Dried red **chillies** and crushed dried red **chillies**

Couscous (Green days only)

Haricot beans (Green days only)

Lentils, all varieties (Green days only)

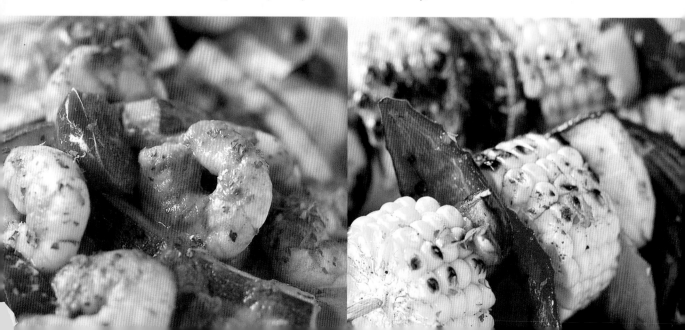

Noodles, all varieties, dried (Green days only)

Pasta, all types, dried (Green days only)

Rice: all varieties, e.g. Basmati, long grain, brown, wild (Green days only)

Passata, plain and flavoured

Bovril stock, all varieties

Vegemite

Tabasco sauce

Fish sauce

Vinegars: e.g. balsamic, red wine, white wine, raspberry

Soy sauces, dark and light

Worcestershire sauce

Fry Light

Spice rack of **ground** and **whole spices**, e.g. Cajun spice seasoning, curry powder, ground cardamom, cinnamon, cloves, coriander, cumin, ground ginger, mustard powder, nutmeg, oregano, paprika, peppercorns, tandoori powder

Mixed **dried herbs**: all varieties

ON THE KITCHEN WORKTOP
Eggs
Garlic
Lemons and **limes**
Onions and **shallots**
Tomatoes, all kinds

FOR THE FRIDGE
Very low-fat natural fromage frais
Very low-fat natural yogurt
Very low-fat natural cottage cheese
Quark soft cheese
Quorn sausages, mince, pieces
Lean **bacon** rashers (Original days only)
Turkey rashers (Original days only)
Caviare and **salmon roe** (Original days only)
Chillies, red and green
Ginger, fresh root
Fresh **herbs**, e.g. basil, bayleaf, chives, coriander, dill, lemongrass, mint, parsley (standard and flat-leaf), rosemary, sage, thyme

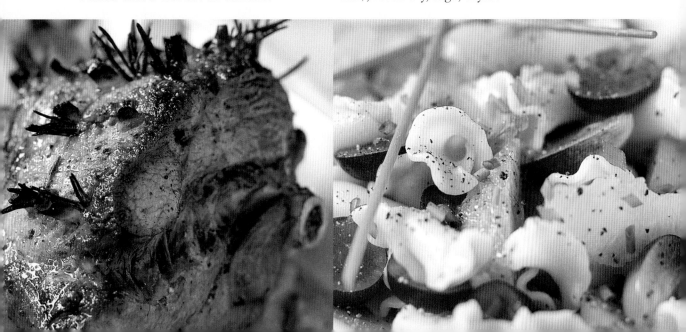

SOUPS

—

STARTERS

MINTED GREEN PEA AND BASIL SOUP

A gorgeous colour and a crunchy–smooth texture with a tang of herbs make a lovely fresh soup.

serves 4   preparation time **10 minutes**   cooking time **30 minutes**

3 large shallots, finely chopped

1 garlic clove, peeled and finely chopped

4 tbsp chopped basil leaves

4 tbsp chopped mint leaves

900ml/1½ pints chicken stock made from Bovril

500g/1lb 2oz frozen or fresh peas

salt and freshly ground black pepper

to serve

very low-fat natural yogurt

to garnish

mint and basil leaves

Place the shallots in a medium saucepan with the garlic and chopped herbs. Pour over the stock, bring to the boil, cover, reduce the heat to medium and simmer for 10 minutes or until the shallots are tender.

Add the peas, bring back to the boil and cook gently for 5 minutes. Season well to taste.

Transfer half the mixture to a food processor and blend until smooth. Return to the pan with the remaining soup and stir to mix well.

Ladle the soup into bowls and serve with a swirl of the yogurt. Garnish with mint and basil leaves and serve immediately.

Green: **Free**

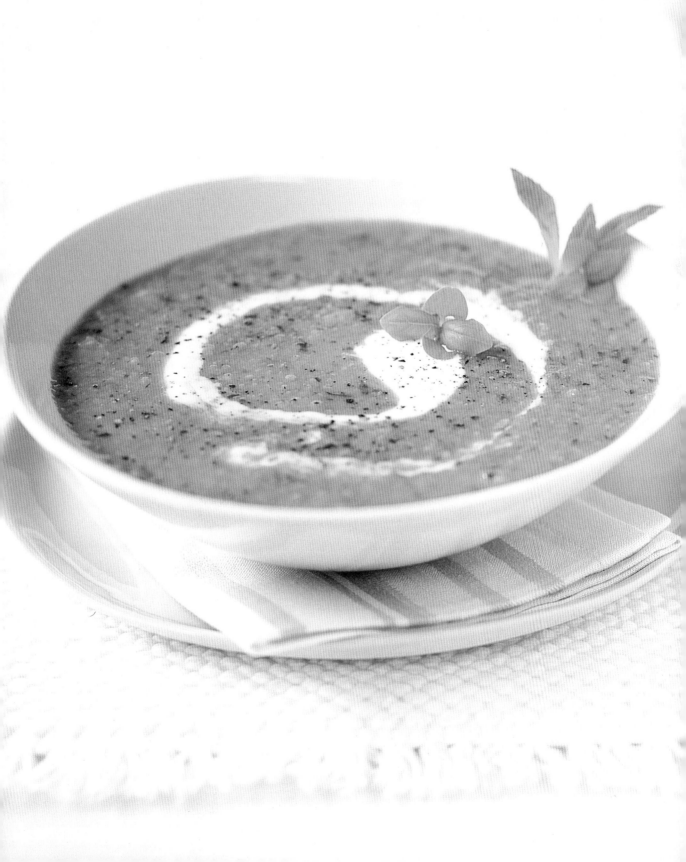

ROASTED YELLOW PEPPER SOUP

A super-healthy soup, ideal for a summer lunch. Don't worry about the amount of garlic; it adds a rich depth to the flavour when cooked.

serves 4 preparation time **10 minutes** cooking time **50 minutes**

6 large yellow peppers

10 ripe plum tomatoes

6 whole garlic cloves

2 tbsp light soy sauce

2 tbsp chopped basil leaves

salt and freshly ground black pepper

to garnish

basil leaves

Preheat the oven to 200°C/Gas 6. Halve and deseed the peppers and place on a non-stick baking sheet and roast for 15 minutes.

Halve the tomatoes and add to the peppers with the garlic cloves and roast for a further 25–30 minutes.

Remove from the oven and carefully peel the skin off the peppers and discard. Place the peeled peppers in a food processor with the tomatoes. Squeeze the garlic from their skins into the processor with the soy sauce and chopped basil leaves. Add 300ml/12fl oz hot water and process until smooth.

Transfer the mixture to a saucepan and place over a medium heat. Bring to the boil, remove from the heat and season well before serving, ladled into warmed soup plates or bowls and garnished with the basil leaves.

Green/Original: **Free**

COURGETTE AND TOMATO SOUP

This soup is very quick to make yet looks really impressive served with swirls of creamy-tasting yogurt.

serves 4 preparation time **20 minutes** cooking time **12 minutes**

1 large onion, peeled

4 courgettes

1 litre/1³/₄ pints chicken stock made from Bovril

4 tbsp chopped mint leaves

to serve

100g/4oz very low-fat natural yogurt

salt and freshly ground black pepper

Finely chop the onion and place in a saucepan. Coarsely grate the courgettes and add to the onion. Stir in the stock and bring the mixture to the boil. Cover, reduce the heat and cook gently for 6–8 minutes.

Transfer half the mixture to a food processor with the mint leaves and blend until smooth. Return the blended mixture to the saucepan with the remaining soup and stir to mix well.

To serve, heat the soup until hot, remove from the heat and stir in the yogurt. Season well and ladle into warmed bowls.

SWEETCORN AND CORIANDER SOUP

The pasta shapes and sweetcorn make this a really substantial soup, and fresh coriander adds a burst of colour and flavour.

serves 4   preparation time **10 minutes**   cooking time **25 minutes**

Fry Light for spraying

8 spring onions, trimmed and finely sliced

1 garlic clove, peeled and crushed

900ml/1½ pints chicken stock made from Bovril

2 x 400g/14oz cans sweetcorn niblets

½ red pepper, deseeded and very finely diced

50g/2oz dried mini pasta shapes

a large handful of fresh coriander leaves, finely chopped

salt and freshly ground black pepper

Spray a large non-stick saucepan with Fry Light and place over a medium heat. Add the spring onions and garlic and stir-fry for 1–2 minutes.

Pour in the stock, increase the heat to high and add the sweetcorn and red pepper. Bring the mixture to the boil, cover and cook for 10 minutes.

Add the pasta, re-cover and let simmer for 10 minutes. Stir in the chopped coriander, season well and remove from the heat. Ladle into warmed bowls and serve immediately.

Green: **Free**

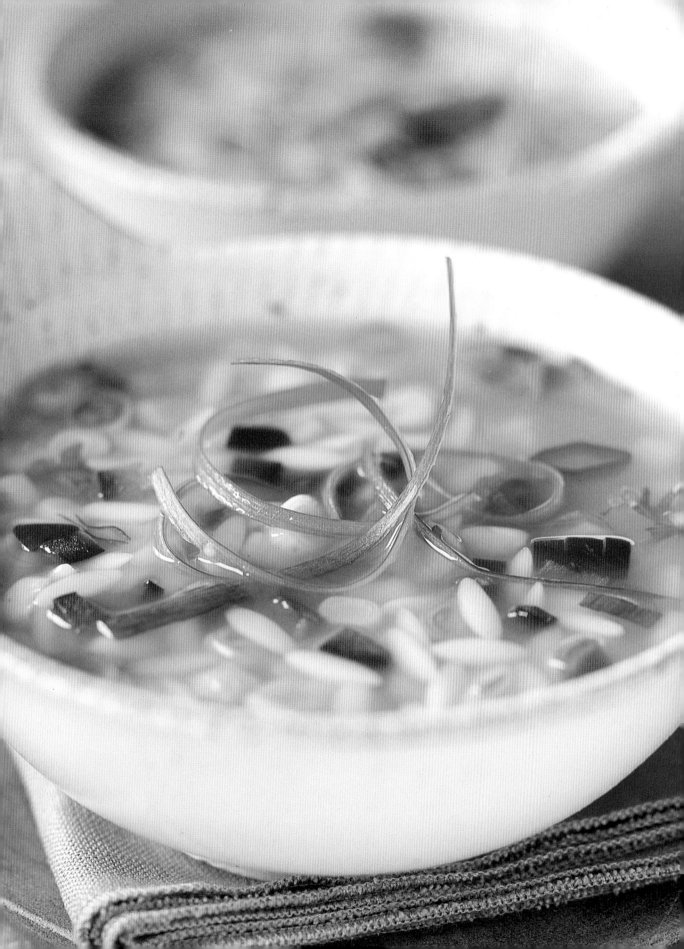

RICH ONION SOUP

A real winter warmer! Slow-cooking the onions gives a deep sweetness to the flavour that blends wonderfully with the savoury beef stock.

serves 4 preparation time **15 minutes** cooking time **1 hour 40 minutes**

600g/1lb 6oz large onions, peeled

2 garlic cloves, peeled

Fry Light for spraying

a few sprigs of thyme

1.5 litres/2½ pints beef stock made
   from Bovril

1 tbsp artificial sweetener

salt and freshly ground black pepper

to serve

very low-fat natural fromage frais

Halve the onions and slice them very thinly. Finely slice the garlic. Spray a non-stick saucepan with Fry Light and place over a medium heat. Add the onions and garlic and stir and cook for 6–8 minutes before turning the heat to low. Allow to cook gently for about 35–40 minutes, stirring occasionally until the onions are lightly browned. Add the thyme sprigs and stir and cook for 2–3 minutes.

Pour in the beef stock and bring to the boil. Cover, reduce the heat to low and simmer gently for 40–45 minutes, stirring occasionally. Add the sweetener and season well.

To serve, ladle the soup into warmed bowls and stir in a spoonful of the fromage frais. Eat immediately.

Green/Original: **Free**

BARLEY SCOTCH BROTH

This is a tasty, traditional soup, just like Mum used to make. The nourishing barley with vegetables is comfort food at its best.

Serves 4 preparation time **20 minutes** cooking time **1 hour 15 minutes**

100g/4oz pearl barley

1 onion, peeled

2 carrots, peeled

4 celery sticks

1 garlic clove

Fry Light for spraying

1 bay leaf

1 x 400g/14oz can chopped tomatoes

1 litre/1³/₄ pints chicken stock made from Bovril

1 tbsp artificial sweetener

4 tbsp chopped flat-leaf parsley

salt and freshly ground black pepper

Place the barley in a large pan of lightly salted water and bring to the boil.

Reduce the heat to medium and cook for 35–40 minutes. Drain and set aside.

Meanwhile, finely dice the onion, carrot and celery and finely chop the garlic. Spray a non-stick saucepan with Fry Light and place over a medium heat. Add the onion, carrots, celery, garlic and bay leaf and stir and cook for 6–8 minutes.

Stir in the tomatoes, stock and sweetener and bring to the boil. Add the drained barley and cook gently for 20–25 minutes. Stir in the chopped parsley, season well and serve ladled into warmed bowls or soup plates.

ITALIAN-STYLE STUFFED PEACHES

A sophisticated starter that's made in minutes; one taste is enough to transport you to the Tuscan hills!

serves 4 preparation time **15 minutes**

4 ripe peaches

150g/5oz very low-fat natural fromage frais

50g/2oz Quark soft cheese

1 tsp very finely grated lemon zest

2 tsp lemon juice

4 tbsp very finely chopped mixed herbs

salt and freshly ground black pepper

to garnish

finely grated lemon zest

Using a sharp knife, cut the peaches in half lengthways and carefully remove the stones.

Place the peaches on a serving platter or plate, cut side up.

In a small bowl, whisk the fromage frais and Quark until smooth and then stir in the lemon zest and juice and chopped herbs, reserving some for garnishing, and mix well to combine. Season to taste.

Spoon this herby mixture into the centre of the peaches. Garnish with the reserved chopped herbs and grated lemon zest and serve immediately.

Green/Original: **Free**

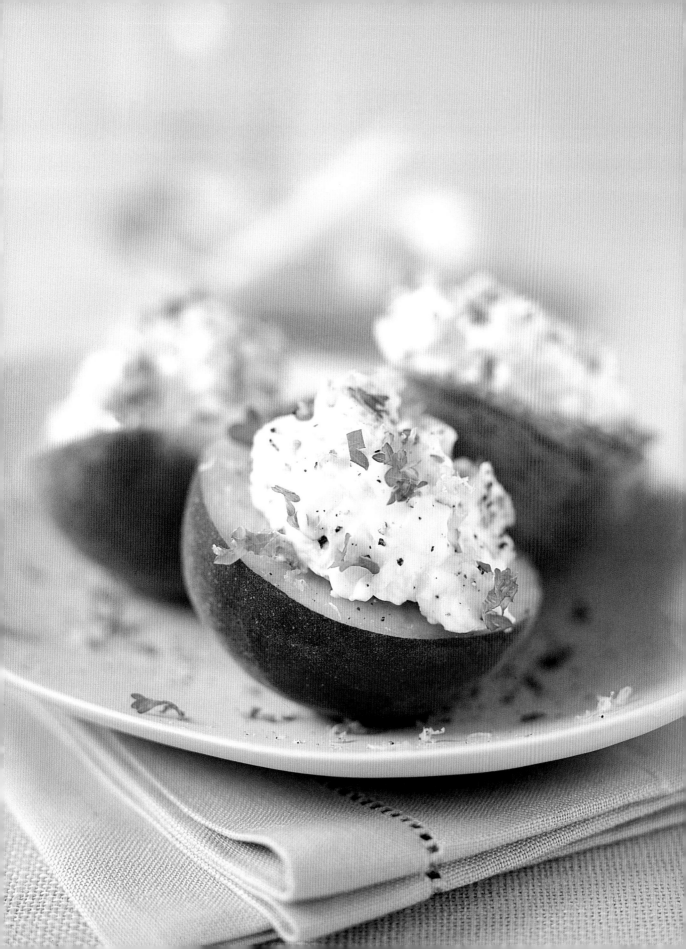

BAKED STUFFED PEPPERS

You could serve this very tasty dish as a lunch with a green salad, or as an accompaniment to a pasta bake or veggie burgers for a substantial and delicious Green day supper.

serves 4   preparation time **20 minutes**   cooking time **25 minutes**

4 large red peppers, halved and
   deseeded
6 spring onions, finely sliced
2 garlic cloves, peeled and crushed
2 ripe plum tomatoes, roughly chopped

200g/7oz cooked Basmati rice
1 x 400g/14oz can red kidney beans in
   chilli sauce
2 tbsp finely chopped flat-leaf parsley
salt and freshly ground black pepper

Preheat the oven to 200°C/Gas 6. Place the peppers cut side up on a non-stick baking sheet.

In a large mixing bowl, mix together the spring onions, garlic and tomatoes.

Stir in the cooked rice, kidney beans and chopped parsley and season well.

Carefully divide this mixture between the pepper halves. Cover loosely with foil and bake in the oven for 20–25 minutes. Serve immediately with a crisp green salad.

Green: **Free**

RICE AND HERB CAKE

This is a really original and moreish dish that can be made ahead – ideal for summer entertaining, picnics or just for nibbling on when you're peckish!

serves 4   preparation time **20 minutes**   cooking time **20 minutes**

500g/1lb 2oz cooked Thai jasmine rice

Fry Light for spraying

1 red chilli, deseeded and finely
  chopped

8 spring onions, trimmed and thinly
  sliced

8 tbsp finely chopped mixed fresh
  herbs (coriander, mint and dill)

4 large eggs

salt

Place the rice in a mixing bowl and set aside.

Spray a medium-sized, non-stick frying pan with Fry Light and place over a medium heat. Add the red chilli to the pan with the spring onions. Stir and cook for 3–4 minutes and then transfer to the rice. Stir to mix well and then add the herbs and continue to combine until evenly mixed.

Beat the eggs and add to the rice mixture and season with salt. Mix well.

Spray the frying pan again with Fry Light and place over a medium heat. Spoon the rice mixture into the pan, patting down to compress and levelling the surface. Cook gently for 6–8 minutes and then place the pan under a medium grill and cook for 6–8 minutes until the cake is set. Remove from the grill and allow to cool completely. To serve, cut the cake into wedges and accompany with a tomato salad.

CUMIN-SCENTED CHICKPEA FALAFELS

Middle Eastern spices such as cumin and ginger add a fragrant lightness to these chunky, savoury, bite-sized burgers. Great for parties or for serving with couscous and roasted vegetables as a main meal.

serves 4 preparation time **20 minutes + chilling** cooking time **20 minutes**

1 onion, peeled and finely chopped

1 carrot, peeled and coarsely grated

2 x 400g/14oz can chickpeas, rinsed and drained

2 garlic cloves, peeled and finely chopped

1 tsp finely grated ginger

2 tsp ground cumin

1 tsp chilli powder

1 tsp ground coriander

3 tbsp very finely chopped fresh coriander

1 small egg

salt

Fry Light for spraying

to serve

very low-fat natural yogurt

Place the onion, carrot, chickpeas, garlic, ginger, cumin, chilli powder and the ground and fresh coriander in a food processor. Pulse and process for 1–2 minutes or until blended but still fairly chunky in texture.

Transfer the mixture to a mixing bowl. Lightly beat the egg and add to the mixture. Season with salt and, using your fingers, mix thoroughly to combine. Cover and chill in the fridge for 6–8 hours to firm up and allow the flavours to develop.

Preheat the oven to 200°C/Gas 6. Line a large baking sheet with non-stick baking parchment and spray lightly with Fry Light. Shape the chickpea mixture into bite-sized balls and place on the prepared baking sheet. Spray lightly with Fry Light and cook in the oven for 15–20 minutes or until lightly golden and firm. Serve warm, with the yogurt to dip into.

Green: **Free**

MIXED GRILLED BALSAMIC PEPPERS

Roasting peppers is worth the effort as it brings out their full colour and sweetness; the balsamic vinegar adds a delicious tang.

serves 4   preparation time **20 minutes + standing**   cooking time **15 minutes**

4 yellow peppers

4 red peppers

2 orange peppers

1 garlic clove, peeled and crushed

2 tbsp balsamic vinegar

salt and freshly ground black pepper

a handful of fresh basil leaves

to serve

red endive or radicchio leaves

Halve and deseed the peppers and place on a foil-lined grill rack, cut side down. Heat a grill to medium–high and place the peppers under it. Cook for 12–15 minutes or until the skins are charred and blackened. Remove from the grill and place in a large plastic bag. Set aside for 10 minutes.

When cool enough to handle, carefully peel the skins off the peppers, discarding the skins but saving any of the juices in a bowl. Cut the pepper into strips and add to the bowl with the crushed garlic and balsamic vinegar. Season and toss to mix well. Cover and let stand at room temperature for 30 minutes for the flavours to develop.

To serve, arrange a few red endive or radicchio leaves on the base of four serving plates. Toss the basil in with the peppers and divide the mixture between the four plates. Serve immediately.

SMOKED TROUT PARCELS

These pretty pink and green parcels are easy to make ahead for a light dinner party starter; the secret ingredient is the lime zest, which gives an extra-fresh zing. Add a little caviare for a super-luxurious touch!

serves 4   preparation time **20 minutes**

100g/4oz Quark soft cheese

2 tbsp very finely chopped dill

2 tbsp very finely snipped chives

1 tsp very finely grated lime zest

1 garlic clove, peeled and crushed

salt and freshly ground black pepper

8 x 25g/1oz slices smoked trout

long chives

to garnish

very low-fat natural fromage frais

salmon roe or caviare

dill sprigs

Place the Quark in a small bowl. Add the chopped dill and chives with the lime zest and garlic. Season and mix well to combine.

Lay the smoked trout slices on a clean work surface and spoon the Quark mixture into the centre of each one. Carefully roll up the slices to form neat parcels and, using long chives, tie up the parcels to form 'presents'. Chill until ready to serve and then place small spoonfuls of fromage frais on top of each parcel and garnish with salmon roe or caviare and sprigs of dill.

Original: **Free**

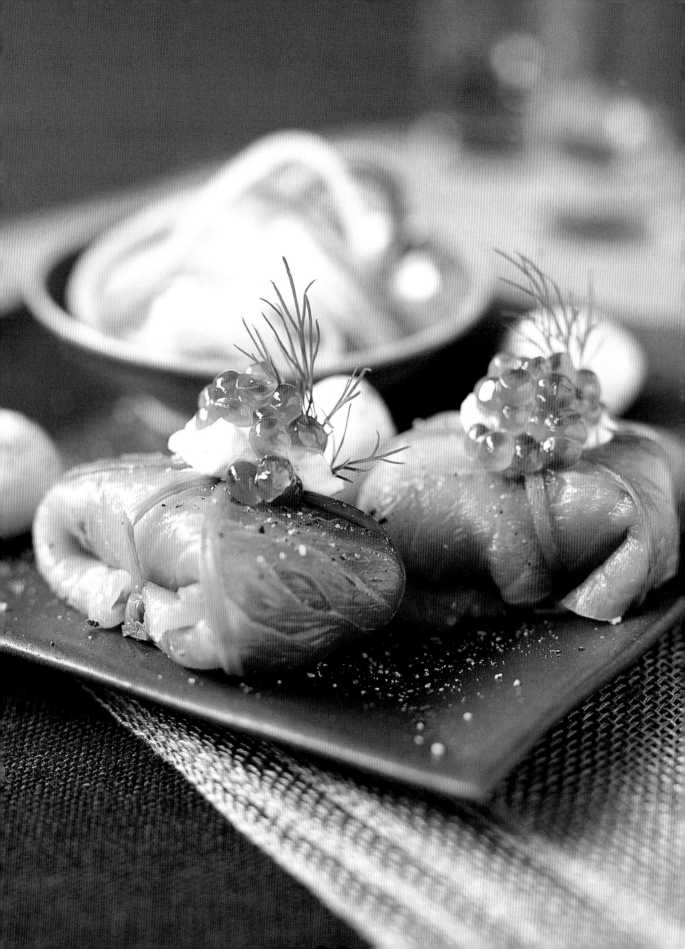

HAM AND PINEAPPLE STICKS

The sweet and sour sauce brings this classic canapé recipe bang up to date.
Everyone will love it!

serves 4   preparation time **20 minutes**

for the sauce
3 tbsp raspberry vinegar
2 tbsp artificial sweetener
1 x 200g/7oz can chopped tomatoes
1 garlic clove, peeled and crushed
salt and freshly ground black pepper

for the sticks
1 x 450g/1lb can lean ham
½ ripe pineapple
2 spring onions

To make the sauce, place the vinegar, sweetener, tomatoes and garlic in a food processor. Blend until smooth, season well and transfer to a small bowl. Chill until ready to use.

Cut the ham into 32 bite-sized pieces. Cut the skin off the pineapple, core and cut the pineapple into 32 bite-sized pieces. Cut the spring onions into eight 2.5cm/1in lengths.

Carefully thread four pieces of ham and four pieces of pineapple alternately onto eight long bamboo skewers, finishing off each skewer with a piece of spring onion. Serve the ham and pineapple sticks with the sweet and sour sauce to dip into.

Original: Free

PRAWN, CHIVE AND PORK BAKED DUMPLINGS

Make lots of these Thai-flavoured mini meatballs as they will disappear as soon as you take them out of the oven. The fresh flavours and meaty texture are a winning combination.

serves 4 preparation time **10 minutes + chilling** cooking time **20 minutes**

250g/9oz extra lean minced pork

250g/9oz raw tiger prawns

8 spring onions, trimmed and very
  finely chopped

6 tbsp very finely snipped chives

2 garlic cloves, peeled and crushed

1 tsp finely grated ginger

1 tbsp soy sauce

1 tbsp very finely chopped lemongrass

1 green chilli, deseeded and very finely
  chopped

salt

Fry Light for spraying

to serve

light soy sauce

Place the pork in a food processor. Using a sharp knife, chop the prawns roughly and add to the pork. Add the spring onions, chives, garlic, ginger, soy, lemongrass and green chilli. Season well with salt and process until fairly smooth. Transfer to a bowl, cover and chill overnight.

Preheat the oven to 200°C/Gas 6. Line a large baking sheet with non-stick baking parchment. Using wet hands, divide the pork mixture into about 20 portions and shape each one into a ball. Place on the prepared baking sheet and spray lightly with Fry Light.

Bake in the oven for 15–20 minutes or until cooked through. Serve hot with a little bowl of light soy sauce for dipping into.

TUSCAN SARDINE PÂTÉ
WITH **VEGETABLE CRUDITÉS**

Whip up a home-made sardine pâté in minutes – served with chunky vegetable sticks it makes a very healthy starter or snack.

serves 4 preparation time **15 minutes + chilling**

2 x 120g/4½ oz cans sardines in
   tomato sauce
250g/9oz Quark soft cheese
finely grated zest and juice of 1 lemon
salt and freshly ground black pepper
2 tbsp capers

6 tbsp finely chopped flat-leaf parsley
for the crudités
1 large carrot
4 celery sticks
1 red pepper

Place the sardines in a mixing bowl. Add the Quark and, using a fork, stir to combine. Add the lemon zest and juice and stir to mix well. Season.

Rinse and drain the capers and add to the sardine mixture together with the chopped parsley. Mix the ingredients together until fairly well combined. Alternatively, for a smoother pâté, place all the ingredients in a food processor and blend until smooth.

Transfer the pâté to a serving bowl or a couple of individual ramekins, cover with cling film and allow to chill in the fridge for 3–4 hours to let the flavours steadily develop.

Meanwhile, peel the carrots and cut them and the celery into dipping-size sticks. Deseed the red pepper and cut into thick strips. To serve, place the sardine pâté on a platter surrounded by the vegetable crudités.

Original: Free

CHICKEN AND VEGETABLE SKEWERS

The longer you can marinate the chicken pieces in the mildly spiced, creamy marinade, the more they will absorb the flavours to make a tender, tangy contrast with the juicy tomatoes.

serves 4 preparation time **10 minutes + marinating** cooking time **15 minutes**

4 large chicken breast fillets, skinned

2 tbsp mild curry powder

150g/5oz very low-fat natural yogurt

juice of 2 limes

1 tbsp artificial sweetener

2 tsp cumin seeds

300g/11oz cherry tomatoes

to serve

salt and freshly ground black pepper

lime wedges

Cut the chicken into bite-sized pieces and place in a non-reactive bowl. Mix together the curry powder, yogurt, lime juice, sweetener and cumin seeds. Pour this mixture over the chicken and toss to coat evenly. Cover and marinate in the fridge for 6–8 hours or overnight if time permits.

Preheat the oven to 220°C/Gas 7 and line a large baking sheet with non-stick baking parchment.

Thread the chicken alternately with the cherry tomatoes onto eight long metal skewers. Place the skewers onto the prepared baking sheet and place in the oven and cook for 12–15 minutes or until the chicken is cooked through. To serve, season well and squeeze over wedges of lime before eating.

SNACKS

ROASTED STUFFED AUBERGINES

A classic flavouring of cinnamon and coriander brings out the full smoky sweetness of roasted aubergine, and the couscous and chickpeas make this a very satisfying meal.

serves 4 preparation time **20 minutes** cooking time **40 minutes**

100g/4oz couscous

2 medium aubergines

6 spring onions, trimmed and finely sliced

4 tbsp chopped coriander leaves

2 plum tomatoes, finely chopped

1 x 400g/14oz can chickpeas, drained

1 tsp ground cinnamon

salt and freshly ground black pepper

Preheat the oven to 220°C/Gas 7. Place the couscous in a heatproof bowl and pour over enough boiling water to only just cover. Cover and leave to stand for 10 minutes. Fluff up the couscous grains with a fork and set aside.

Meanwhile, halve the aubergines lengthways and, using a sharp-edged teaspoon, carefully scoop out the aubergine flesh from the centre, leaving the skin intact to form a shell. Finely chop the scooped out flesh and mix into the prepared couscous with the spring onions, coriander leaves, tomatoes, chickpeas and cinnamon. Season well.

Pack the couscous mixture into each aubergine shell. Place on a non-stick baking sheet, cover with foil and place in the oven and roast for 25 minutes. Remove the foil and cook for a further 10–15 minutes or until the aubergines have collapsed slightly and are tender. Serve immediately with a crisp green salad if desired.

Green: Free

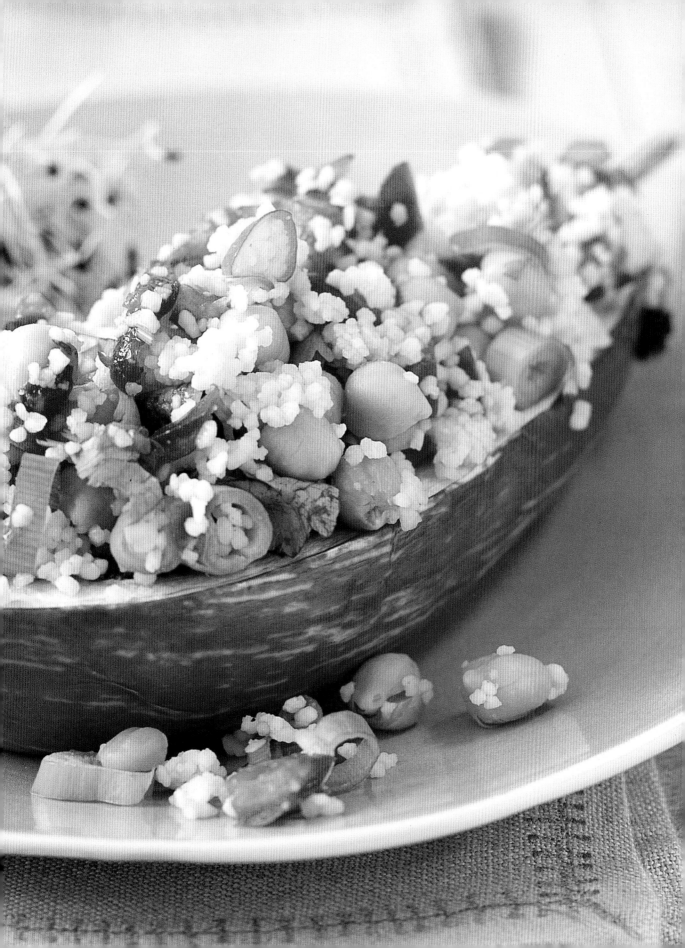

HERB PANCAKES WITH CAJUN-STYLE BEAN SALSA

A dish that combines the influences of northern Europe and the Deep South with great results. Start preparing the potato pancake mix well in advance.

serves 4 preparation time **20 minutes + chilling** cooking time **25 minutes**

1kg/2lb 4oz potatoes (Desirée)
1 onion, peeled and finely chopped
150ml/5fl oz chicken stock made
   from Bovril
6 tbsp finely chopped coriander
1 large egg
salt and freshly ground black pepper
Fry Light for spraying
for the salsa
1 x 200g/7oz can baked beans in
   tomato sauce

1 x 200g/7oz can red kidney beans,
   rinsed and drained
1 x 200g/7oz can sweetcorn kernels,
   rinsed and drained
4 spring onions, trimmed and very
   finely sliced
1 plum tomato, roughly chopped
1 red chilli, deseeded and very finely
   chopped
3 tbsp very finely chopped mint leaves
salt

Peel the potatoes and roughly chop. Place in a saucepan of salted water and bring to the boil. Simmer for 10–12 minutes. Drain and return to pan.

Place the onion in a small saucepan with the stock and bring to the boil. Reduce the heat, cover and simmer for 4–5 minutes or until tender. Add the onion to the potato and mash well. Allow to cool and then add the chopped coriander. Lightly beat the egg and add to the potato mixture. Season well and mix thoroughly. Cover and chill for 3–4 hours.

Meanwhile, make the salsa by combining all the ingredients in a bowl. Season well and set aside.

Divide the potato mixture into eight portions and form into pancakes about 12mm/^{1}/$_2$in thick. Lightly spray a non-stick frying pan with Fry Light and heat until hot. Cook the pancakes in batches of two to three, cooking for 2–3 minutes on each side or until golden. Remove to a non-stick baking sheet and keep warm while you cook the rest. Serve with the salsa spooned over.

Green: Free

GARLIC AND CHILLI DIP WITH CRISPY POTATO SKINS

Perfect for a 'big night in' for entertaining, or just when you deserve a comfort-food snack. The cool, creamy dip makes a fantastic contrast with the hot, crispy potatoes.

serves 4 preparation time **15 minutes** cooking time **1 hour 5 minutes**

for the potato skins

4 jacket potatoes

Fry Light for spraying

sea salt

for the dip

250g/9oz very low-fat natural
    fromage frais

4 garlic cloves, peeled and crushed

2 red chillies, deseeded and very finely
    chopped

2 tsp lemon juice

3 tbsp finely chopped dill

2 tbsp chopped parsley

salt

Preheat the oven to 200°C/Gas 6. Prick the potatoes all over with a skewer or prongs of a fork and place on a non-stick baking sheet. Spray with Fry Light and sprinkle over some sea salt. Bake in the oven for 1 hour or until the centres of the potatoes are tender.

Remove from the oven, cut the potatoes in half and, using a spoon, scoop out most of the flesh and save for another recipe, leaving a thin layer of potato around the inside of each shell. Using a sharp knife, cut the potato halves into half again, making 16 potato skins. Place back onto the baking sheet and return to the oven for 5 minutes.

Meanwhile, make the dip by combining all the ingredients in a small bowl and mixing well. Remove the potato skins from the oven and serve immediately with the garlic, dill and chilli dip.

SWEETCORN AND VEGETABLE SKEWERS

An unusual spicy marinade brings out the flavour of colourful grilled vegetables. It's ideal to cook on the barbecue or under the grill if the weather's not so good.

serves 4   preparation time **20 minutes**   cooking time **10 minutes**

2 large courgettes, thickly sliced

1 orange pepper, deseeded and cut into
   bite-sized pieces

1 red pepper, deseeded and cut into
   bite-sized pieces

2 whole sweetcorns, thickly sliced

2 red onions, peeled and cut into
   wedges

4 garlic cloves, peeled and crushed

juice of 2 lemons

1 tsp paprika

handful of flat-leaf parsley, chopped

salt and freshly ground black pepper

Fry Light for spraying

Place the courgettes in a large, shallow, non-reactive bowl. Add the peppers, sweetcorn and onion wedges.

Mix together the garlic, lemon juice and paprika and pour over the vegetable mixture. Toss to coat evenly. Add the chopped parsley, season well and thread the vegetables alternately onto eight metal skewers.

Spray each skewer with Fry Light and then place under a hot grill or on a barbecue and cook for 5–10 minutes, turning often, until the vegetables are cooked through, tender and lightly charred. Serve immediately with a crisp salad, couscous or steamed rice.

Green: Free

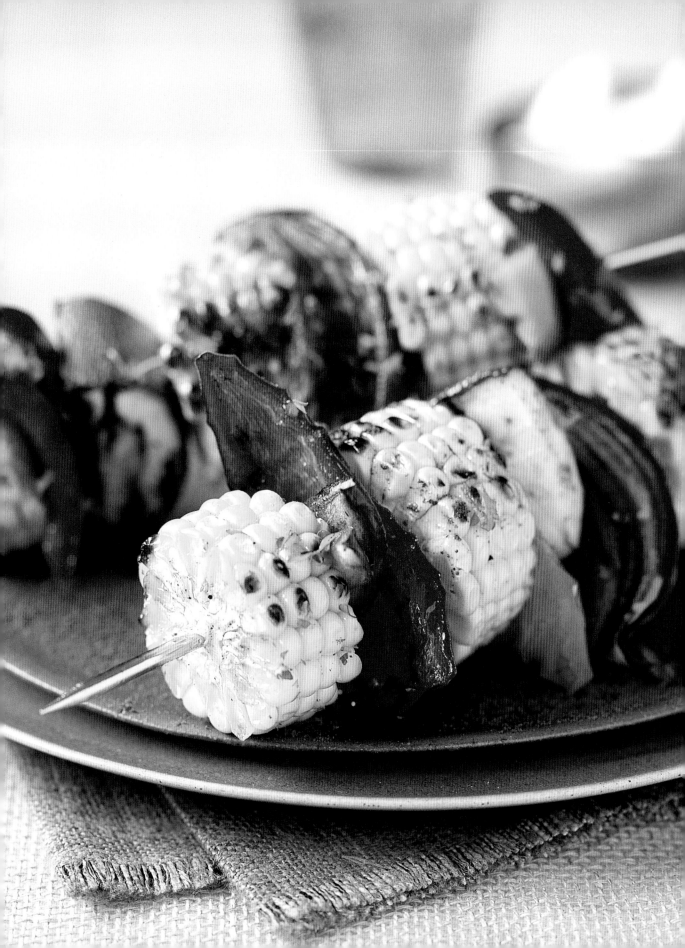

POTATO AND MUSHROOM JACKETS

This creamy mushroom filling propels the 'boring old baked potato' into a different league. Once the potatoes are cooked, the filling is quickly made.

serves 4   preparation time **20 minutes**   cooking time **1 hour 10 minutes**

4 jacket potatoes

Fry Light for spraying

300g/11oz chestnut mushrooms

2 garlic cloves, peeled and crushed

2 spring onions, trimmed and finely
 sliced

75ml/2¹/₂fl oz chicken stock made
 from Bovril

salt and freshly ground black pepper

10 tbsp very low-fat natural fromage
 frais

3 tbsp very finely chopped chives

2 tbsp chopped flat-leaf parsley

Preheat the oven to 220°C/Gas 7. Place the potatoes on a non-stick baking sheet and prick all over with the prongs of a fork. Spray each one with Fry Light and place in the oven and cook for about 1 hour or until tender in the centre. Remove from the oven.

Meanwhile, wipe and roughly chop the mushrooms and place in a non-stick frying pan with the garlic, spring onions and the stock. Place over a high heat and cook rapidly, stirring often, for 6–8 minutes. Season well.

Halve the potatoes lengthways and scoop out the flesh and transfer to a mixing bowl. Stir in the fromage frais and chives, season and mix well to combine. Spoon this mixture back into the scooped out potato shells and top each one with the mushroom mixture. Sprinkle over the parsley and serve immediately with a green salad.

Green: Free

CHIPS AND A DIP

Yes, you can have chips when you're slimming! These home-made, low-fat chips are Free on Green days and taste just great served as a snack with a tasty, chunky vegetable dip.

serves 4   preparation time **20 minutes**   cooking time **30 minutes**

for the chips

5–6 large waxy potatoes (Maris Piper)

Fry Light for spraying

sea salt

for the dip

1 x 100g/4oz can chopped tomatoes

50g/2oz bottled or canned roasted red
   peppers, drained

2 garlic cloves, peeled and crushed

½ small cucumber, diced

3 tbsp red wine vinegar

200g/7oz very low-fat natural fromage
   frais

1 tsp artificial sweetener

salt and freshly ground black pepper

Preheat the oven to 200°C/Gas 6. Bring a large saucepan of lightly salted water to the boil. Peel and cut the potatoes into thick chips and place in the saucepan. Boil for 3–4 minutes and then drain thoroughly. Return to the saucepan, cover with a lid and shake the pan gently to rough up the edges; this helps in creating a crisp coating when baked.

Line a large baking sheet with non-stick baking parchment and spray it with Fry Light. Spread the chips in a single layer and re-spray with Fry Light. Sprinkle over some sea salt and bake in the oven for 15–20 minutes, turning the chips halfway through.

While the chips are cooking, make the dip by placing all the ingredients in a food processor. Blend until smooth, season well and transfer to a small bowl. Chill until ready to serve with the warm chips.

STUFFED TOMATO SALAD

It looks really impressive, but this is a no-cook lunch or supper that's easily made with storecupboard ingredients and some tasty fresh vegetables.

serves 4 preparation time **20 minutes**

4 large, ripe beefsteak tomatoes

1 small red onion, peeled and finely
   diced

1 small cucumber, finely diced

1 small yellow pepper, finely diced

2 tbsp finely chopped wild rocket
   leaves

1 x 200g/7oz can tuna in water,
   drained

1 tbsp capers, sliced

2 tbsp fat-free vinaigrette-style dressing

juice of 1 lemon

salt and freshly ground black pepper

Cut the tops off the tomatoes and carefully hollow them out, using a small teaspoon. Discard the seeds of the tomatoes and roughly dice the flesh and place in a bowl with the red onion, cucumber, yellow pepper and rocket, reserving some of the chopped rocket leaves for garnishing.

Flake the tuna into the vegetable mixture and add the capers. Mix together the dressing and lemon juice, season well, stir into the salad mixture and toss to combine.

Carefully spoon this mixture back into the tomato 'shells' and serve immediately topped with the remaining rocket leaves.

Original: Free

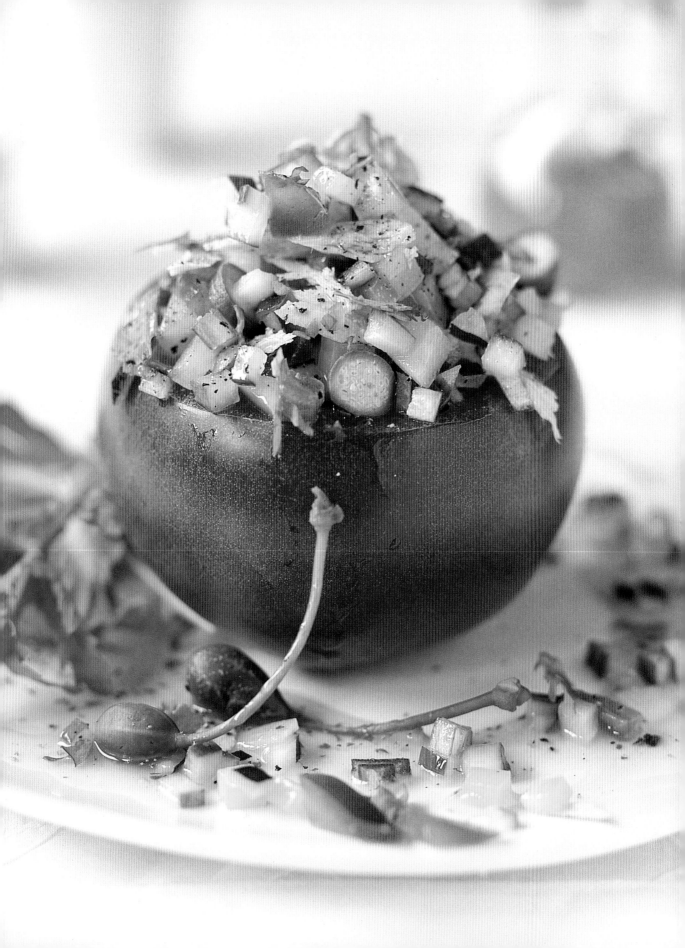

SWEET AND SPICY WEDGES WITH CUCUMBER RAITA

'Chips and a dip' with a super exotic twist! Sweet potatoes make delicious, tender chips and the paprika and cumin bring out their full flavour.

serves 4   preparation time **10 minutes**   cooking time **25 minutes**

Fry Light for spraying
6 large sweet potatoes
1 tbsp sweet smoked paprika
1 tsp ground cumin
1 tbsp sea salt
juice of 2 lemons

for the raita
1/2 small cucumber
200g/7oz very low-fat natural yogurt
5 tbsp very finely chopped mint leaves
salt and freshly ground black pepper

Preheat the oven to 200°C/Gas 6. Line a large baking sheet with non-stick baking parchment and spray it lightly with Fry Light.

Wash and scrub the sweet potatoes and then cut them into thick wedges. Arrange them on the prepared baking sheet.

In a small bowl, mix together the paprika, cumin, salt and the lemon juice and brush this mixture onto the wedges. Spray with Fry Light and place in the oven and cook for 20–25 minutes or until just tender and lightly golden.

While the sweet potatoes are cooking, make the raita by coarsely grating the cucumber into a bowl. Squeeze out any excess liquid, stir in the yogurt and mint leaves and season well. Serve the sweet and spicy wedges with the raita.

Green: Free

STUFFED CHICKEN AND COURGETTE 'SANDWICH'

This is a chicken Kiev with a difference; the creamy, savoury filling and juicy courgette make an irresistible combination of textures and flavours for a light but very satisfying dish.

serves 4 preparation time **20 minutes** cooking time **15 minutes**

4 large chicken breast fillets, skinned

200g/7oz Quark soft cheese

2 garlic cloves, peeled and crushed

1 tbsp very finely chopped tarragon

1 tsp very finely grated lemon zest

salt and freshly ground black pepper

1 large courgette, thinly sliced

Fry Light for spraying

Sandwich each chicken breast with cling film and place on a clean work surface. Using a wooden mallet, gently beat the breast until it is almost doubled in size and very thin (being careful not to break the flesh). Cut each chicken portion into two fairly equal-sized pieces.

In a bowl, mix together the Quark, garlic, tarragon and lemon zest and season well to taste.

Preheat the oven to 200°C/Gas 6 and line a large baking sheet with non-stick baking parchment.

Carefully spread the Quark mixture on top of all the chicken pieces with a palette knife. Lay four chicken pieces, Quark side up, on the prepared baking sheet, well spaced. Divide the sliced courgettes between the four pieces to cover neatly. Top each portion with the remaining chicken pieces, Quark side down, to form a 'sandwich'.

Using cocktail sticks, skewer the pieces together, season well and spray with Fry Light. Place in the oven and cook for 12–15 minutes or until the chicken is cooked through and the centre is oozing. Serve immediately with a crisp lettuce and tomato salad.

CHICKEN AND HERB BALLS

The mixture of herbs and spices in these bite-sized chicken balls ensures that each one just bursts with flavour – fantastic to serve at parties or with pre-dinner drinks.

serves 4   preparation time **10 minutes + chilling**   cooking time **20 minutes**

4 spring onions, trimmed and very
   finely chopped
2 garlic cloves, peeled and crushed
500g/1lb 2oz lean chicken mince
1 red chilli, deseeded and very finely
   chopped
1 tsp ground ginger
1 tsp ground cumin

1 tsp ground coriander
2 tbsp very finely chopped coriander
   leaves
2 tbsp very finely chopped mint leaves
salt and freshly ground black pepper
to serve
lime wedges

Place the spring onions, garlic, chicken mince, red chilli, ground spices and chopped herbs into a mixing bowl. Season and, using your fingers, mix thoroughly. Cover and chill for 3–4 hours.

Preheat the oven to 200°C/Gas 6. Line a large baking sheet with non-stick baking parchment.

Divide the mixture into 16 portions and then shape each portion into a ball. Place the balls on the prepared baking sheet and place in the oven for 20 minutes or until cooked through. Remove from the oven and serve hot, accompanied with a fresh tomato salsa (see page 90) or a very low-fat natural fromage frais dip, if desired, and lime wedges.

Original: **Free**

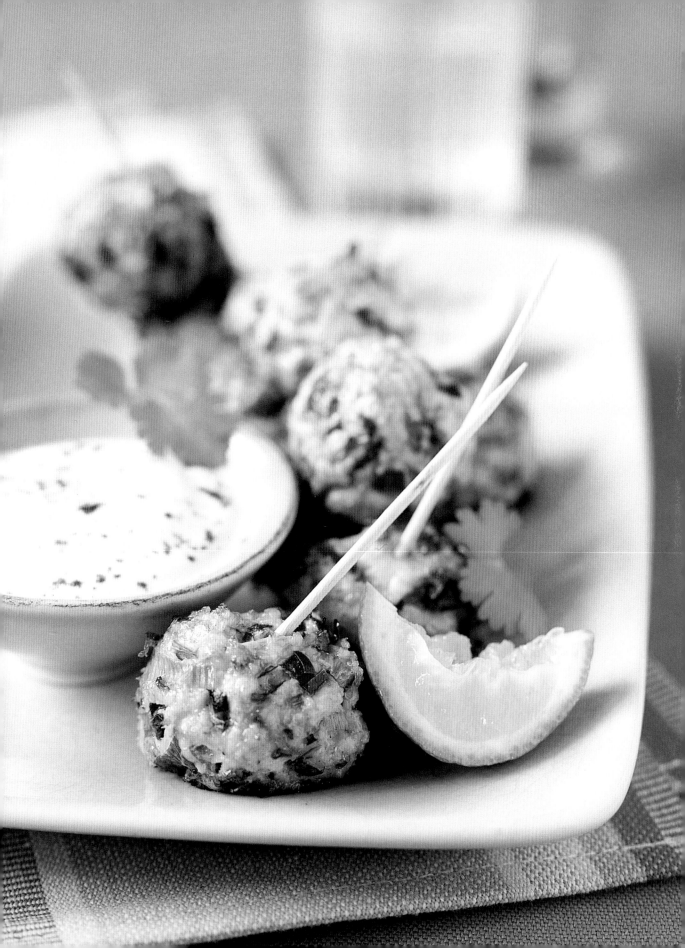

GLAMORGAN SAUSAGES
WITH TOMATO SAUCE

These vegetarian 'sausages' are bound to be a hit with meat-lovers too; serve them with a tasty tomato sauce and fresh vegetables for a very filling supper.

serves 4 preparation time **20 minutes + chilling** cooking time **20 minutes**

for the sauce
250ml/9fl oz passata with herbs
1 tbsp balsamic vinegar
1 tbsp Worcestershire sauce
1 tbsp artificial sweetener
salt and freshly ground black pepper

for the sausages
1 x 400g/14oz can cannellini beans
1 red onion, peeled and very finely
 diced
6 tbsp very finely chopped parsley
2 carrots
1 tsp dried mixed herbs
a dash of Tabasco sauce
salt and freshly ground black pepper
Fry Light for spraying

To make the sauce, place the passata in a small saucepan with the balsamic vinegar, Worcestershire sauce, sweetener and seasoning. Bring to the boil, cover and simmer very gently for 4–5 minutes, stirring often. Set aside to cool.

Rinse and drain the beans and place in a food processor with the onion and parsley. Grate in the carrots and add the dried mixed herbs and Tabasco sauce. Season and pulse to combine. Remove the mixture from the processor and transfer to a mixing bowl. Cover and chill in the fridge for 3–4 hours.

When ready to cook, preheat the oven to 200°C/Gas 6. Line a large baking sheet with non-stick baking parchment. Divide the bean mixture into eight portions and form each into a sausage shape about 6–7.5cm/2^{1}/$_{2}$–3in long.

Place on the prepared baking sheet and spray with Fry Light. Place in the oven and cook for 10–12 minutes or until browned. Carefully remove from the oven onto warmed plates and serve immediately with the tomato sauce.

Green: Free

BANGERS AND MASH

Amazingly, this version of bangers and mash is Free on both Green and Original days. If you haven't tried pumpkin and celeriac mash, give it a go – it's a great alternative to potato.

serves 4 preparation time **20 minutes** cooking time **1 hour**

for the mash
700g/1lb 9oz pumpkin
700g/1lb 9oz celeriac
2 tsp thyme leaves
4 spring onions, trimmed and very
  finely sliced
4 tbsp very low-fat natural fromage
  frais
salt and freshly ground black pepper

for the bangers
8 Quorn sausages
Fry Light for spraying
for the gravy
6 large shallots, finely sliced
200ml/7fl oz chicken stock made from
  Bovril

Peel the pumpkin and discard the seeds. Roughly chop and place in a large saucepan. Peel the celeriac, roughly chop and place with the pumpkin in the saucepan. Pour over water and bring to the boil. Reduce the heat and simmer gently for 15–20 minutes or until the vegetables are tender. Drain and return to the pan.

Using a potato masher, mash the vegetables until fairly smooth and stir in the thyme leaves, spring onions and fromage frais. Season, set aside and keep warm.

Meanwhile, preheat the oven to 200°C/Gas 6. Place the sausages on a non-stick baking sheet, spray with Fry Light and cook for 20–25 minutes or until cooked through.

While the sausages are cooking make the gravy by cooking the shallots with the stock in a small saucepan. Bring to the boil, reduce the heat and cook for 10–12 minutes, stirring often until the shallots are tender.

Place two sausages on each of four warmed plates and serve with the mash. Spoon over the shallot gravy and eat immediately.

SNACKS

SPICY PORK BURGERS

Replace the bread with meaty, flat mushrooms and you have a burger that's Free on Original days. And these are burgers with a kick – serve with a fresh, cooling salad to delight spice-lovers everywhere.

serves 4 preparation time **20 minutes + chilling** cooking time **20 minutes**

100g/4oz fine green beans
1 red onion
700g/1lb 9oz lean pork mince
1 tbsp hot curry powder
salt

8 large, flat mushrooms
Fry Light for spraying
to serve
slices of tomato, cucumber and onion

Cut the beans into 1cm/½in lengths and blanch for 2–3 minutes in lightly salted boiling water. Drain and transfer to a mixing bowl. Peel and chop the onion finely and add to the beans with the pork mince and curry powder. Season well with salt. Using your fingers, mix well to combine thoroughly then cover and chill for 1–2 hours.

Preheat the oven to 200°C/Gas 6. Line a large baking sheet with non-stick baking parchment. Divide the pork mixture into eight portions and form each one into a burger. Place on the baking sheet.

Remove the stalks from the mushrooms and place, gill side up, on the baking sheet. Season and lightly spray the burgers and the mushrooms with Fry Light. Place in the oven and cook for 12–15 minutes or until the burgers are cooked through and the mushrooms are very tender.

To serve, place two mushrooms on each serving plate and top with the burgers. Top each burger with slices of tomato, cucumber and onion and serve immediately.

Original: Free

PASTRAMI HASH POTS

Whoever said cottage cheese was boring? Here it's teamed with celeriac and pastrami to create a very tasty and substantial bake that's perfect for a weekend lunch.

serves 4   preparation time **20 minutes**   cooking time **25 minutes**

200g/7oz celeriac, peeled

100g/4oz very low-fat natural cottage
   cheese

200g/7oz pastrami

3 large eggs, lightly beaten

2 spring onions, trimmed and finely
   chopped

2 tbsp passata with herbs

2 tbsp finely chopped flat-leaf parsley

salt and freshly ground black pepper

Cut the celeriac into 1cm/½in cubes and place in a saucepan of boiling water. Cook for 2–3 minutes and then drain.

Place the cottage cheese in a mixing bowl. Roughly chop the pastrami into small pieces and add to the cheese with the eggs, spring onion, celeriac and passata. Stir in the chopped herbs and season well.

Preheat the oven to 200°C/Gas 6. Spoon the mixture into four individual ramekins or gratin dishes. Place in the oven and cook for 20 minutes or until set and golden on the top. Remove from the oven and serve immediately.

MEAT
—
POULTRY

GRIDDLED CHICKEN AND TOMATO SALSA

Chicken breasts can be a bit bland – but not if you spritz them with lime juice, grill them until they're tender and juicy, and serve them with a tangy salsa with a spicy kick.

serves 4 preparation time **15 minutes**   cooking time **20 minutes**

for the salsa

4 ripe plum tomatoes, finely chopped

1 green chilli, deseeded and finely
  sliced

1 red onion, peeled and finely chopped

a large handful of flat-leaf parsley,
  chopped

salt and freshly ground black pepper

for the chicken

4 boneless, skinless chicken breasts

juice of 1 lime

salt and freshly ground black pepper

Fry Light for spraying

to serve

lime wedges

To make the salsa, combine all the ingredients in a bowl, stir to mix well and season. Cover and set aside.

Sprinkle the chicken with the lime juice and season well. Spray each breast with Fry Light.

Heat a non-stick griddle pan over a medium heat and cook the chicken for 8–10 minutes on each side or until cooked through.

Remove from the heat and place onto warmed plates. Spoon over the salsa and serve immediately with a crisp green salad and lime wedges.

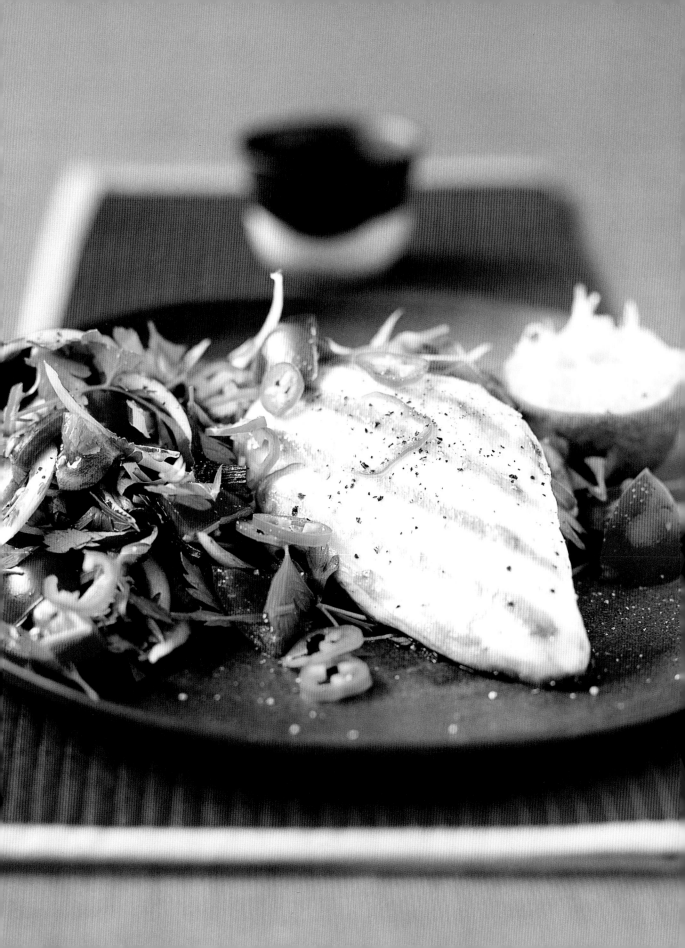

MEDITERRANEAN CHICKEN HOT POT

Slow-cooking the chicken and vegetables in this casserole creates a deliciously fragrant, meltingly tender dish that will become an instant 'all-time favourite'.

serves 4   preparation time **20 minutes** cooking time **1 hour 45 minutes**

6 large chicken breast fillets, skinned

1 x 400g/14oz can tomatoes

3 garlic cloves, peeled and finely chopped

6 shallots

1 red pepper

1 yellow pepper

2 courgettes

200g/7oz mushrooms

1 tsp dried mixed herbs

1 tbsp artificial sweetener

700ml/23fl oz chicken stock made from Bovril

salt and freshly ground black pepper

to serve

a large handful of fresh basil leaves

Preheat the oven to 200°C/Gas 6. Cut the chicken into bite-sized pieces and place in a medium casserole dish with the canned tomatoes.

Add the garlic to the chicken mixture. Halve and peel the shallots, deseed the peppers and cut into bite-sized pieces and add to the casserole dish.

Thickly slice the courgettes and mushrooms and add to the chicken mixture with the dried mixed herbs, artificial sweetener and chicken stock. Place the casserole dish over a high heat and bring to the boil. Cover very tightly and place in the oven and cook for 1½ hours.

Remove from the oven, season well and stir in the fresh basil leaves just before serving.

SWEET AND SOUR CHICKEN

Enjoy the flavours of sweet and sour chicken without the sticky heaviness of a restaurant version – it's just as quick as a takeaway too.

serves 4 preparation time **15 minutes + marinating** cooking time **10 minutes**

6 chicken breast fillets, skinned

6 spring onions, trimmed and finely sliced

2 garlic cloves, peeled and finely chopped

salt and freshly ground black pepper

3 tbsp light soy sauce

Fry Light for spraying

1 tbsp dark soy sauce

2 tbsp artificial sweetener

2 tbsp raspberry vinegar

1 tsp paprika

1/2 tsp Chinese five-spice powder

100ml/31/2fl oz passata

Slice the chicken very thinly and place in a shallow, non-reactive dish. Sprinkle over the spring onions and garlic, season well and pour over the soy sauce. Toss to mix well, cover and marinate in the fridge for 30 minutes.

Spray a large, non-stick frying pan with Fry Light and, when hot, add the chicken mixture and cook over a high heat. Stir and cook for 5–6 minutes and then add the dark soy, sweetener, vinegar, paprika, Chinese five-spice and passata. Stir to mix well and bring the mixture to the boil.

Reduce the heat and cook gently for 3–4 minutes or until the chicken is cooked through. Check seasoning and serve immediately.

CHICKEN TIKKA MASALA

Your local Indian restaurant will wonder what's happened to you once you've discovered this fantastic home-made version of a classic dish that's Free on Original days.

serves 4   preparation time **20 minutes**   cooking time **25 minutes**

4 chicken breast fillets, skinned

Fry Light for spraying

salt and freshly ground black pepper

2 large shallots, peeled

3 garlic cloves, peeled

½ tsp crushed cardamom seeds

½ tsp turmeric

1 tbsp tikka masala powder or
   tandoori spice blend powder

4 tbsp passata

150ml/5fl oz stock made from Bovril

100g/4oz very low-fat natural fromage
   frais

to serve

very low-fat natural fromage frais

chopped fresh coriander

lime wedges (optional)

Spray the chicken with Fry Light, season and place under a hot grill and cook for 15–16 minutes, turning once until cooked through. Remove and, when cool, cut into bite-sized pieces. Set aside.

Using a fine grater, grate the shallots and garlic into a bowl.

Spray a large non-stick frying pan with Fry Light and place over a medium heat. Add the shallot and garlic mixture with the crushed cardamom seeds, turmeric and tikka masala powder. Stir-fry for 1 minute before adding passata.

Add the chicken and stock and cook for 4–5 minutes, stirring often. Add the fromage frais, season to taste and remove from the heat. Drizzle over a little fromage frais, garnish with chopped coriander and lime wedges, if desired, and serve with steamed cabbage or any other Free vegetables of your choice.

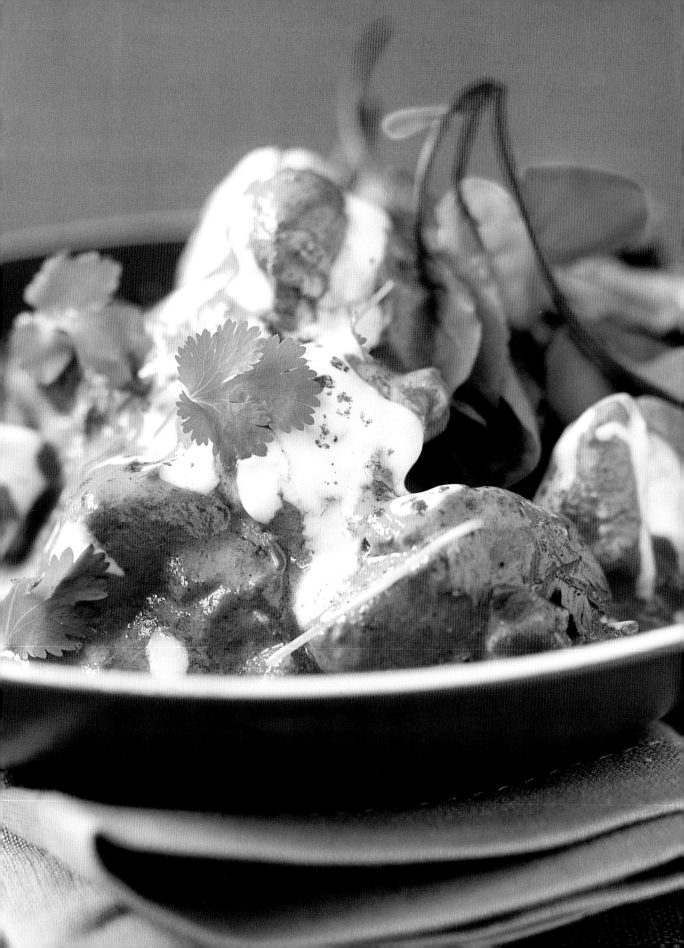

TURKEY PESTO ROAST

Pesto sauce can be very high in Syns; our lighter version has just as much flavour and is a perfect partner for tasty, meaty turkey steaks. Marinate the turkey for as long as possible for the best results.

serves 4 preparation time **20 minutes + marinating** cooking time **25 minutes**

for the pesto

3 garlic cloves, peeled

8 tbsp very finely chopped basil leaves

4 tbsp very finely chopped parsley

2 tbsp balsamic vinegar

1 tbsp Worcestershire sauce

8 tbsp chicken stock made from Bovril

salt and freshly ground black pepper

for the turkey roast

4 turkey steaks

Fry Light for spraying

to garnish

basil leaves

To make the pesto, finely grate the garlic and place it in a food processor with the basil and parsley. Add the balsamic vinegar, Worcestershire sauce and stock and blitz until fairly smooth. Add a little more stock if the mixture is too thick to process smoothly. (You will need to use a small food processor as the quantities are too little for a regular-sized one.) Season and transfer to a bowl.

Place the turkey steaks in a single layer in a shallow, non-reactive dish and spread over the pesto. Coat evenly, cover and allow to marinate in the fridge for 3–4 hours, or overnight, if time permits.

Preheat the oven to 200°C/Gas 6 and line a large baking sheet with non-stick baking parchment. Place the turkey steaks on the prepared baking sheet and spray with Fry Light. Place in the oven and roast for 20–25 minutes or until cooked through. Serve immediately garnished with basil leaves.

GRILLED TANDOORI DUCK

Giving duck a spicy tandoori coating complements the richness of the meat very well and tenderises it too. So when you grill it, it will have a melt-in-the-mouth texture.

serves 4   preparation time **10 minutes + marinating**   cooking time **15 minutes**

4 boneless, skinless duck breasts

salt and freshly ground black pepper

8 tbsp very low-fat natural yogurt

2 tbsp tandoori spice blend powder

2 garlic cloves, peeled and crushed

2 tsp finely grated ginger

juice of 1 lemon

1 tbsp artificial sweetener

6 tbsp passata

to serve

chopped fresh coriander and mint
  leaves

Place the duck breasts on a clean work surface and, using a short, sharp knife, make three or four diagonal slits in each breast. Season the breasts well and place in a single layer in a shallow, non-reactive dish.

In a small bowl, mix together the yogurt, tandoori spice blend, garlic cloves, ginger, lemon juice, sweetener and passata. Pour this mixture over the duck and toss to coat evenly. Cover and marinate in the fridge overnight for the flavours to develop.

To cook, preheat a grill to medium–high. Place the duck breasts on a foil-lined grill rack and place about 7–8cm/3–3½in under the grill. Cook for 5–6 minutes on each side or until cooked to your liking. Serve immediately, garnished with the coriander and mint leaves and serve with a chopped tomato and cucumber salad.

MUSTARD AND GARLIC-ROASTED LEG OF LAMB

Rosemary is a classic flavouring for roast lamb, and here it receives a further boost with mustard and garlic. Perfect for a special Sunday lunch.

serves 4–6 preparation time **15 minutes** cooking time **1 hour 30 minutes + resting**

1 small leg of lamb, weighing about 3kg/6lb 12oz and trimmed of all visible fat

3 tbsp mustard powder

10 garlic cloves, peeled

rosemary sprigs

sea salt and freshly ground black pepper

Preheat the oven to 230°C/Gas 8.

Rub the leg of lamb all over with the mustard powder. Cut each garlic clove into 3–4 long slivers and, using a short sharp knife, stud the flesh of the lamb all over with the garlic and small sprigs of rosemary. Season liberally with salt and freshly ground black pepper.

Place in a roasting tin and put in the oven for 10–12 minutes per 500g/1lb for rare lamb or 15 minutes per 500g/1lb for medium. But after the first 15 minutes reduce the heat to 180°C/Gas 4. Baste the meat from time to time with the pan juices.

When ready, remove from the oven and allow the lamb to rest, covered in foil, in a warm place for 15–20 minutes before carving and serving.

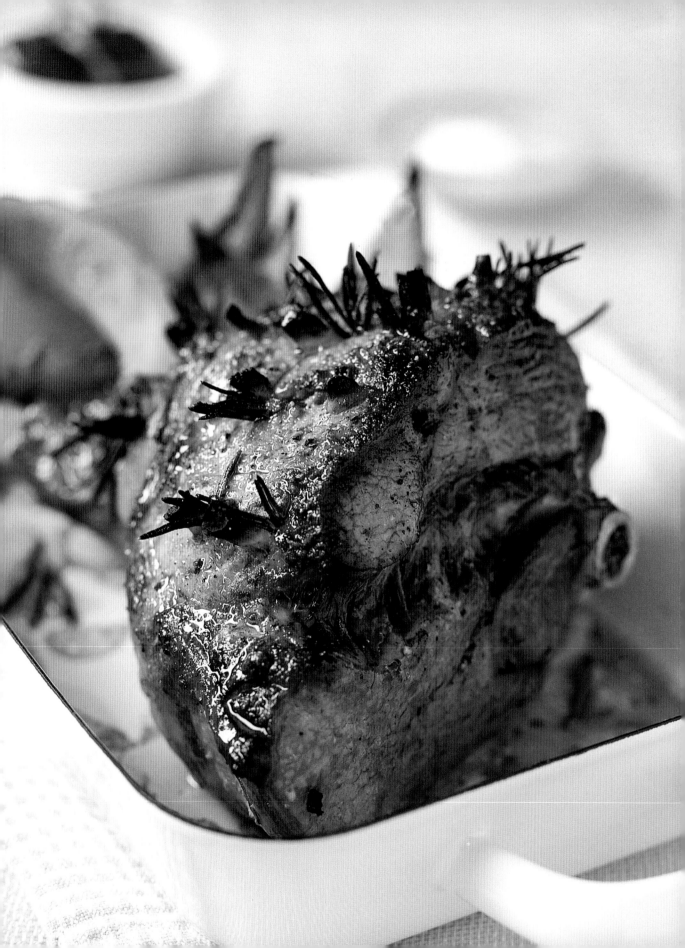

ROSEMARY LAMB STEAKS WITH MINT AND TOMATO CHUTNEY

Lamb steaks are great for midweek suppers as they're quick to cook and very satisfying. Marinate the lamb and make the chutney the night before so that it's on the table in minutes when you get home.

serves 4   preparation time **15 minutes + marinating**   cooking time **30 minutes**

4 lean lamb steaks, trimmed of all
   visible fat
1 tbsp very finely chopped rosemary
   leaves
2 garlic cloves, peeled and crushed
100g/4oz very low-fat natural yogurt
freshly ground black pepper
Fry Light for spraying

for the chutney
1 x 400g/14oz can chopped tomatoes
½ red onion, peeled and finely
   chopped
2 tbsp artificial sweetener
salt
a large handful of chopped mint leaves

Place the lamb steaks in a shallow, non-reactive dish in a single layer. In a small bowl, mix together the rosemary leaves, garlic and yogurt. Season liberally with black pepper and mix well. Spread this mixture over the lamb steaks to coat evenly. Cover and marinate for 24 hours.

Meanwhile, make the chutney by placing the tomatoes, onion and sweetener in a small saucepan. Bring to the boil, reduce the heat and cook gently for 15–20 minutes, stirring often. Season well with salt, remove from the heat and stir in the mint leaves.

At the same time, heat a large, non-stick griddle pan until hot. Spray the lamb steaks with Fry Light and cook over a high heat for 4–5 minutes on each side or until cooked to your liking. Serve the steaks immediately accompanied by the chutney.

MOROCCAN LAMB KOFTAS

This is a traditional dish that offers an exotic and delicious mixture of flavours and textures. The sweet sharpness of the lemons blends beautifully with the spices and the richness of the lamb.

serves 4   preparation time **20 minutes**   cooking time **25 minutes**

1 red onion, peeled and finely chopped

1kg/2lb 4oz lean minced lamb

3 tsp ground cumin

2 tsp ground coriander

2 tsp ground cinnamon

2 tsp ground ginger

2 tsp chilli powder

salt and freshly ground black pepper

3 preserved lemons, roughly chopped

700ml/23fl oz chicken stock made from Bovril

to serve

a handful of chopped fresh coriander leaves

Place the onion in a large mixing bowl with the lamb and 1 tsp each of the ground spices. Season well and, using your fingers, mix well to combine. Using wet hands, shape the mixture into walnut-sized balls and set aside.

Place the remaining ground spices in a medium, non-stick saucepan with the preserved lemons and the stock and bring to the boil. Cover tightly, reduce the heat and simmer for 3–4 minutes.

Carefully add the meatballs to the saucepan, cover the pan and let simmer gently for 15–20 minutes, turning them often until cooked through. Check seasoning.

To serve, ladle into four warmed soup plates or bowls and sprinkle over chopped coriander leaves.

CURRIED PORK BROCHETTES
WITH **MANGO SALSA**

A fresh, fruity mango salsa is the ideal accompaniment to these spicy brochettes, which have a double kick of fresh chilli and curry powder.

serves 4   preparation time **20 minutes + chilling**   cooking time **10 minutes**

1 red chilli, deseeded and finely chopped

6 spring onions, trimmed and finely sliced

900g/2lb lean pork mince

2 tbsp medium or hot curry powder

3 tbsp finely chopped mint leaves

50g/2oz very low-fat natural yogurt

finely grated zest and juice of 1 lime

salt and freshly ground black pepper

for the salsa

1 ripe mango, peeled, stoned and finely diced

1 bottled roasted red pepper, drained and finely diced

2 tbsp chopped coriander leaves

2 tbsp chopped mint leaves

Place the chilli, spring onions, pork, curry powder, mint leaves, yogurt and lime zest and juice in a bowl and mix well using your fingers. Season, cover and chill for 2–3 hours in the fridge.

Meanwhile, make the salsa by combining all the ingredients in a bowl, toss to mix well and cover and store in the fridge until ready to serve. If you're using bamboo skewers, put eight of them into a bowl of water to soak.

Preheat the grill to high. Divide the mince mixture into 32 portions and shape each one into a smallish ball. Thread four balls onto each skewer and cook under the preheated grill for 4–5 minutes on each side or until cooked through. Serve immediately accompanied by the salsa.

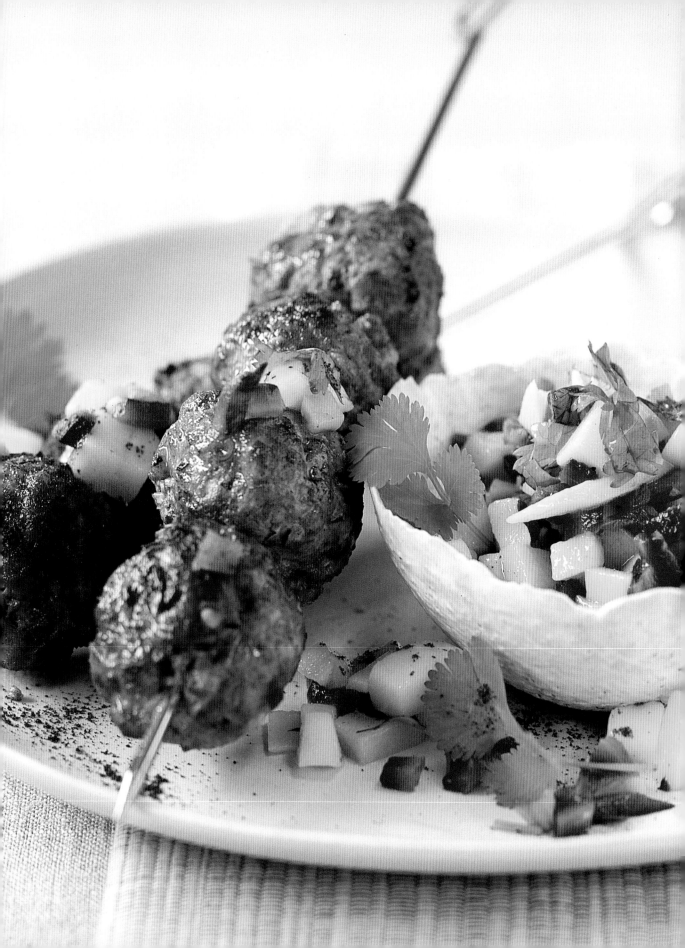

THAI PORK CURRY

Stir-frying is a very quick and healthy way of cooking, and using frozen vegetables in this dish ensures that you have a delicious all-in-one meal that loses none of the fresh, tangy Thai flavours of the spices and sauces.

serves 4 preparation time **15 minutes** cooking time **18 minutes**

500g/1lb 2oz lean pork steaks
Fry Light for spraying
2 garlic cloves, peeled and thinly sliced
1 tbsp very finely chopped lemongrass
1 red chilli, deseeded and thinly sliced
6 spring onions, trimmed and cut into
    4cm/1½in diagonal pieces
1kg/2lb 4oz mixed frozen stir-fry
    vegetables (carrots, onions, peppers,
    broccoli, baby corn, bean sprouts)

200ml/7fl oz chicken stock made from
    Bovril
1 tbsp Thai seven-spice seasoning
4 tbsp soy sauce
1 tbsp fish sauce (optional)
8 tbsp very low-fat natural yogurt
to garnish
chopped sweet basil or coriander
    leaves

Cut away all visible fat from the meat. Place the pork steaks between sheets of cling film and, using a wooden mallet or rolling pin, beat until about 5mm/¼in thick. Cut the pork into very thin strips.

Spray a large non-stick wok or frying pan with Fry Light. Place over a high heat and add the pork strips. Stir-fry for 7–8 minutes or until the pork is sealed, cooked through and lightly browned. Add the garlic, lemongrass, chilli, spring onions and stir-fry over a high heat for 1–2 minutes.

Stir in the frozen vegetables and stir-fry on high for 2–3 minutes. Add the stock, Thai seven-spice seasoning, soy sauce and fish sauce (if using) and stir and cook for 2–3 minutes or until the vegetables are just tender.

Remove from the heat and stir in the yogurt, sprinkle over the fresh herbs and serve immediately.

CREAMY BEEF GOULASH

Smoked paprika gives an extra depth to the spicy flavour of this winter warmer, but standard paprika works well too.

serves 4   preparation time **10 minutes**   cooking time **2 hours**

1 x 400g/14oz can chopped tomatoes

1 large onion, peeled and finely chopped

300g/11oz chestnut mushrooms, sliced

2 red peppers, deseeded and diced

1kg/2lb 4oz lean braising steak, cut into thin strips

2 tbsp smoked Hungarian paprika

½ tsp caraway seeds

1 bay leaf

a pinch of marjoram

1 tsp dried mixed herbs

salt and freshly ground black pepper

250g/9oz very low-fat natural fromage frais

Preheat the oven to 150°C/Gas 2. Put the tomatoes and onion in a saucepan and place over a medium heat. Bring to the boil, reduce the heat and cook gently for 10–12 minutes, until the onions have softened.

Stir in the mushrooms and peppers and cook for a further 6–8 minutes.

Place the steak in an ovenproof casserole dish. Sprinkle over the paprika, caraway seeds, bay leaf, marjoram and dried herbs. Season well and pour over the tomato mixture. Cover tightly and cook in the oven for 1½ hours or until the meat is tender.

Beat the fromage frais until smooth and pour over the casserole before serving. Steamed cabbage and carrots would make a great accompaniment.

CRUSTED FILLET STEAK WITH ROAST VEGETABLE SALSA

The hot, smoky taste of a grilled peppered steak is a perfect match for tender, sweet, roasted Mediterranean vegetables – well worth the time it takes to prepare the peppers, courgette, aubergine and onion.

serves 4   preparation time **25 minutes + marinating**   cooking time **45 minutes**

2 tbsp mixed peppercorns, roughly crushed

1 tbsp Worcestershire sauce

4 fillet steaks, trimmed of all visible fat

for the vegetables

1 red pepper, deseeded and diced

1 yellow pepper, deseeded and diced

1 courgette, trimmed and diced

1/2 aubergine, trimmed and diced

1 red onion, peeled and diced

Fry Light for spraying

salt and freshly ground black pepper

2 tbsp chopped rosemary leaves

Preheat the oven to 200°C/Gas 6. Mix together the crushed peppercorns and the Worcestershire sauce. Spread this mixture over the steaks, cover and allow to marinate for 3–4 hours.

Prepare the vegetables and place on a large roasting tray lined with baking parchment. Spray with Fry Light, season well and sprinkle over the rosemary. Place in the oven and cook for 15–20 minutes or until the vegetables are tender and slightly charred at the edges. Remove and keep warm.

Meanwhile, heat a ridged non-stick griddle pan until hot. Spray the steaks with Fry Light and then cook for 3–4 minutes on each side or until cooked to your liking.

Remove from the pan and allow to rest for 5 minutes before serving with the roasted vegetables. Accompany with steamed green beans, if desired.

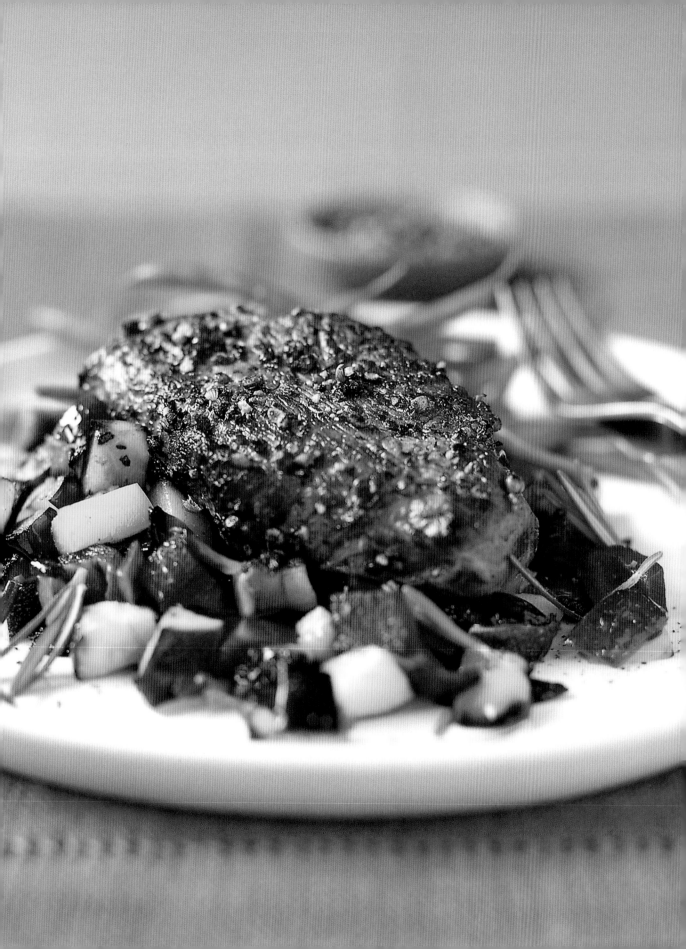

SPICY BEEF AND VEGETABLE STEW

A touch of curry gives an intriguing extra bite to a classic British winter stew of beef and bacon. This is a really 'friendly' dish that will wait happily for you in the oven.

serves 4   preparation time **20 minutes**   cooking time **3 hours 15 minutes**

Fry Light for spraying

2 onions, peeled and finely chopped

800ml/28fl oz beef stock made from Bovril

600g/1lb 6oz lean stewing steak, cut into cubes

4 carrots, peeled and thickly sliced

2 sprigs of thyme

1 bay leaf

1 tbsp medium curry powder

1 leek, cleaned and thinly sliced

2 tbsp chopped parsley

4 rashers of lean bacon, chopped

salt and freshly ground black pepper

Preheat the oven to 160°C/Gas 3. Spray a large non-stick frying pan with Fry Light and add the onions. Stir-fry over a medium heat for 3–4 minutes and then add 4–5 tbsp of the stock and continue to stir and cook for 4–5 minutes or until soft. Transfer to a medium-sized casserole dish and set aside.

Wipe out the frying pan with kitchen paper and re-spray with Fry Light. Place over a high heat and, when hot, add the meat. Stir and fry for 4–5 minutes or until the meat is sealed. Transfer to the casserole dish with any of the pan juices.

Add all the remaining ingredients to the casserole dish, season well, cover tightly and bake in the oven for 3 hours. Remove from the oven, check seasoning and serve immediately.

BEEF, TURNIP AND HERB HOT POT

Garlic and rosemary add fragrance to a rich, juicy stew of beef and tomatoes – and flat-leaf parsley is the perfect finishing touch of colour and peppery flavour.

serves 4 preparation time **15 minutes** cooking time **1 hour 20 minutes**

600g/1lb 6oz lean stewing steak

Fry Light for spraying

2 garlic cloves, peeled and crushed

2 onions, peeled and finely sliced

500g/1lb 2oz turnips, trimmed and cut
  into bite-sized pieces

1 tbsp chopped rosemary leaves

1 bay leaf

2 x 400g/14oz cans chopped tomatoes

2 tbsp beef Bovril

2 tbsp artificial sweetener

salt and freshly ground black pepper

6 tbsp chopped flat-leaf parsley

Trim the steak of all visible fat and cut into bite-sized pieces. Spray a large non-stick saucepan with Fry Light and place over a high heat. Add the meat and stir-fry for 5–6 minutes until sealed and lightly browned. Reduce the heat to medium and add the garlic, onions and turnips. Stir and cook for a further 3–4 minutes.

Add the rosemary and bay leaves to the saucepan with the chopped tomatoes, Bovril and sweetener. Stir well and bring to the boil. Cover tightly, reduce the heat and simmer gently for 1 hour, stirring often.

Season well, remove from the heat and stir in the chopped parsley just before serving.

FISH
DISHES

SEAFOOD AND DILL OMELETTE

An everyday omelette becomes a luxurious treat in minutes with the addition of seafood and a sprinkling of herbs and spices.

serves 4   preparation time **15 minutes**   cooking time **15 minutes**

400g/14oz pack of luxury cooked
    mixed seafood (prawns, squid,
    mussels, etc.)
juice of 1 lemon
4 spring onions, trimmed and thinly
    sliced

salt and freshly ground black pepper
6 large eggs
2 tbsp Worcestershire sauce
4 tbsp finely chopped fresh dill
Fry Light for spraying

Place the seafood in a bowl with the lemon juice and spring onions. Season and toss to mix well.

Place the eggs in a large bowl and lightly beat in the Worcestershire sauce and dill. Season.

Spray a large non-stick frying pan with Fry Light and place over a medium heat. Pour in the eggs and swirl the mixture around to evenly coat the pan. Sprinkle over the seafood mixture onto the surface and reduce the heat, cover and cook gently for 8–10 minutes or until the omelette is just set and the base is golden.

Remove from the heat and serve straight from the pan, cut into wedges and accompanied with a big salad.

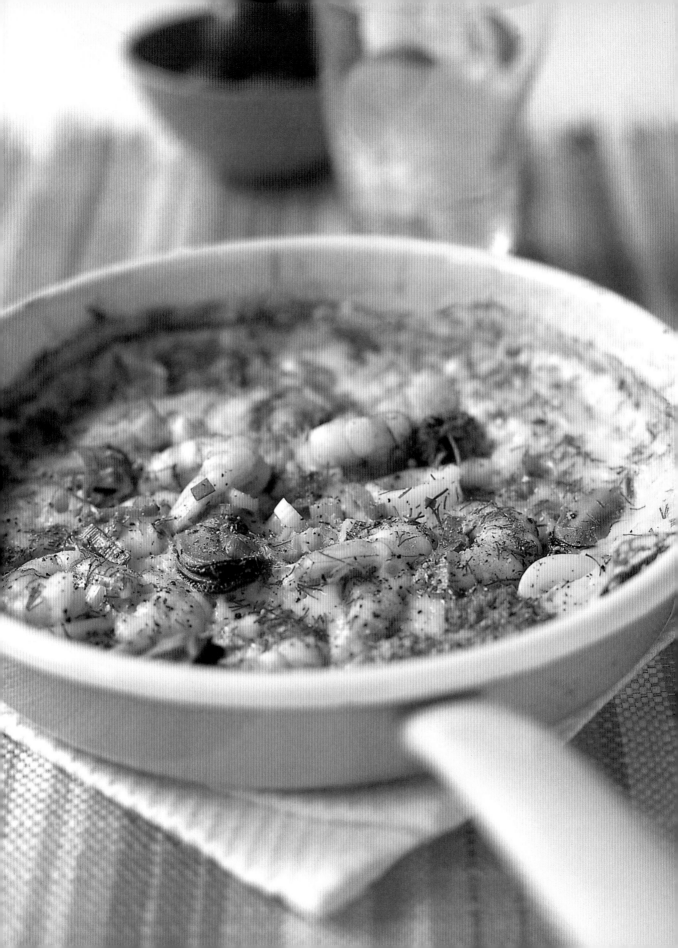

MIXED SEAFOOD STEW

The fennel and spices make this a wonderfully fragrant, sophisticated dish: imagine yourself on a sunny terrace in the south of France!

serves 4 preparation time **15 minutes** cooking time **50 minutes**

1 red pepper, deseeded and roughly chopped

1 leek, trimmed and thickly sliced

1 fennel bulb, trimmed and roughly chopped

2 garlic cloves, peeled and thinly sliced

2 x 400g/14oz cans chopped tomatoes

2 tbsp artificial sweetener

a few drops of Tabasco sauce

600ml/1 pint chicken stock made from Bovril

1 tsp crushed fennel seeds

1 tsp dried mixed herbs

a pinch of saffron threads

1kg/2lb 4oz mixed cooked luxury seafood (prawns, squid, mussels, etc.)

salt and freshly ground black pepper

to garnish

chopped parsley

Place the pepper, leek and fennel pieces in a large non-stick saucepan. Add the garlic together with the tomatoes, sweetener, Tabasco, stock, fennel seeds, mixed herbs and saffron. Place over a high heat and bring to the boil. Reduce the heat, cover tightly and cook gently for 40 minutes, stirring occasionally.

Stir in the cooked seafood, season well and heat through for 3–4 minutes. Remove from the heat and serve immediately, garnished with chopped parsley.

Original: Free

COMFORT FOOD FISH PIE

Take fish pie to the next dimension by adding broccoli and tomatoes along with a generous mixture of fish and a tasty, comforting topping of creamy mashed swede.

serves 4   preparation time **25 minutes**   cooking time **40 minutes**

200g/7oz salmon fillet, skinned

200g/7oz hoki fillet, skinned

Fry Light for spraying

250g/9oz cooked peeled prawns

400g/14oz broccoli florets

2 plum tomatoes, roughly chopped

2 garlic cloves, peeled and crushed

1 egg, beaten

2 tsp mustard powder

2 tbsp Worcestershire sauce

1 tsp Tabasco sauce

4 tbsp chopped chives

4 tbsp chopped flat-leaf parsley

400g/14oz very low-fat natural
   fromage frais

salt and freshly ground black pepper

1kg/2lb 4oz swede, peeled and
   roughly chopped

Preheat the oven to 220°C/Gas 7. Roughly chop the salmon and hoki fillets into bite-sized pieces and place in a frying pan. Pour over water to cover, bring to the boil, cover and simmer for 5 minutes. Remove from the pan with a slotted spoon and place in a Fry Light-sprayed ovenproof dish together with the prawns.

Blanch the broccoli and then drain and add to the fish mixture with the chopped tomatoes.

Mix the garlic with the beaten egg. Mix the mustard powder with 1 tbsp water and add to the egg mixture. Stir in the Worcestershire sauce, Tabasco and chopped herbs. Beat in the fromage frais and season well. Pour this mixture over the fish and toss gently to coat evenly.

Boil the swede in a large pan of lightly salted water and cook for 12–15 minutes until tender. Drain and mash roughly. Spread the swede mash over the fish mixture and place in the oven and cook for 20–25 minutes until hot and bubbling. Serve immediately.

COURGETTE AND PRAWN CURRY

This is a light and colourful curry, ideal for a summer's evening, with lots of juicy flavours and interesting textures – and all cooked in one pan.

serves 4   preparation time **15 minutes**   cooking time **20 minutes**

1 medium onion, peeled and finely
  diced

2 garlic cloves, peeled and crushed

1 tsp finely grated ginger

1 tsp mild chilli powder

2 tsp mild curry powder

200ml/7fl oz chicken stock made with
  Bovril

1 large courgette

6 cherry tomatoes, halved

200ml/7fl oz passata

600g/1lb 6oz cooked, peeled tiger
  prawns

200g/7oz very low-fat natural fromage
  frais

6 tbsp very finely chopped coriander

2 tbsp chopped mint leaves

salt

Place the onion in a medium-sized non-stick saucepan with the garlic, ginger, chilli powder, curry powder and stock. Bring to the boil over a medium heat, cover, reduce the heat to low and cook gently for 3–4 minutes.

Cut the courgette into thick matchsticks and add to the pan with the tomatoes and passata. Bring back to the boil and simmer gently for 10 minutes, stirring often to prevent sticking.

Stir in the prawns, fromage frais and chopped herbs, season with salt and remove from the heat.

Serve immediately with steamed green vegetables and salad.

Original: Free

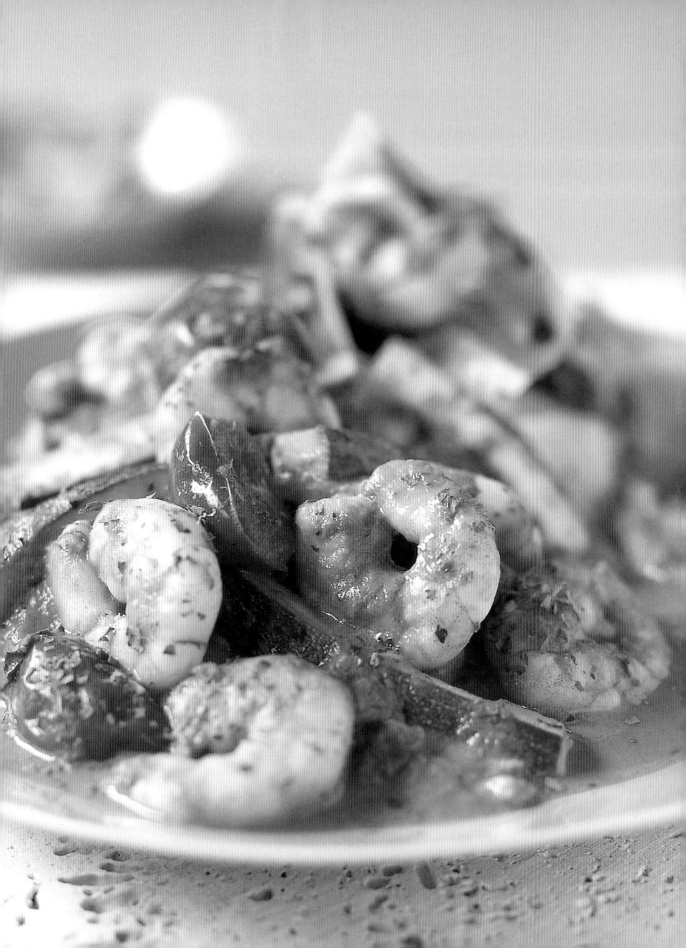

MEXICAN-STYLE PRAWN AND PEPPER STIR-FRY

Cayenne and lime add a hot, fresh flavour to this dish of chunky prawns with sweet, tender peppers and tomatoes.

serves 4   preparation time **15 minutes**   cooking time **25 minutes**

Fry Light for spraying

3 garlic cloves, peeled and thinly sliced

8 spring onions, trimmed and thinly sliced

2 tsp ground cumin

1 tsp cayenne pepper

3 mixed peppers (red, orange and yellow), deseeded and thinly sliced

1 x 400g/14oz can chopped tomatoes

1 tbsp red wine vinegar

150ml/5fl oz chicken stock made from Bovril

2 tbsp artificial sweetener

900g/2lb raw tiger prawns

juice of 1 lime

salt and freshly ground black pepper

Heat a large non-stick wok or frying pan sprayed with Fry Light and place over a medium heat. Add the garlic and spring onion, and stir and cook for 2–3 minutes.

Stir in the ground cumin, cayenne, mixed peppers, tomatoes, red wine vinegar, stock and sweetener. Bring to the boil, reduce the heat and cook for 12–15 minutes, stirring occasionally.

Shell, devein and clean the prawns and add to the tomato mixture. Cook over a high heat for 4–5 minutes or until the prawns turn pink and are just cooked through. Remove from the heat, squeeze over the lime juice, season and serve.

Original: **Free**

COD CAKES WITH TARTARE SAUCE

These are very special fishcakes – made with cod fillet and tiger prawns, and flavoured with a subtle mix of herbs and spices. Using celeriac instead of potato ensures they are Free on Original days.

serves 4 preparation time **20 minutes + chilling** cooking time **30 minutes**

300g/11oz celeriac

2 garlic cloves, peeled and crushed

4 spring onions, trimmed and thinly sliced

a dash of Tabasco sauce

5 tbsp very finely chopped dill

2 tsp finely grated lemon zest

250g/9oz cod fillet, skinned

100g/4oz raw tiger prawns, cleaned

½ small egg, beaten

salt and freshly ground black pepper

Fry Light for spraying

for the tartare sauce

4 small red shallots, very finely diced

2 tbsp capers

4 tbsp chopped gherkins

1 plum tomato, deseeded and roughly chopped

200g/7oz very low-fat natural yogurt

salt and freshly ground black pepper

Peel and cut the celeriac into small pieces and boil in lightly salted water for 8–10 minutes until tender. Drain thoroughly and place in a food processor. Stir in the garlic, spring onions, Tabasco, dill and lemon zest. Roughly chop the cod and the prawns and add to the mixture in the processor with the beaten egg. Season and process until fairly smooth.

Transfer to a bowl, cover and chill for 3–4 hours or overnight for the mixture to firm up and to allow the flavours to develop.

Preheat the oven to 200°C/Gas 6. Line a large baking sheet with non-stick baking parchment. Divide the fish mixture into eight portions and shape each into a ball. Flatten to form 'cakes' and place on the baking sheet. Spray with Fry Light and bake in the oven for 15–20 minutes or until cooked through.

While the cakes are cooking make the sauce by combining all the ingredients in a bowl, season well and chill until ready to serve. Serve the cod cakes warm and spoon over the sauce 'tartare'.

FISH GREEN MASALA

Indian spices complement the fresh taste of cod very well, and the marinade makes a spicy, zesty sauce.

serves 4 preparation time **20 minutes + marinating** cooking time **20 minutes**

4 large, thick cod fillets, skinned

8 tbsp very finely chopped coriander

6 tbsp very finely chopped mint

juice and finely grated zest of 1 lime

2 garlic cloves, peeled and crushed

1 tsp ground ginger

1 green chilli, chopped

1 tbsp artificial sweetener

100ml/3^1/$_2$fl oz chicken stock made
   from Bovril

1 tbsp fish sauce

salt and freshly ground black pepper

Place the cod in a shallow, non-reactive dish in a single layer.

Place the coriander, mint, lime zest and juice, garlic, ginger, green chilli and sweetener in a food processor and pulse for a few seconds. Pour in the stock and fish sauce and blend until fairly thick and smooth, adding a little more stock if necessary. Season well.

Spoon this mixture over the cod and toss to coat well. Cover and allow to marinate in the fridge for 30 minutes.

Preheat the oven to 200°C/Gas 6. Place the fish on a non-stick baking sheet and bake for 15–20 minutes or until the fish is cooked through and flakes easily. Serve warm with a tomato salad.

Original: Free

TOMATO AND MONKFISH KEBABS

The firm flesh of monkfish makes it ideal for adding to colourful kebabs to cook on the barbecue or on the grill.

serves 4   preparation time **15 minutes + marinating**   cooking time **15 minutes**

1kg/2lb 4oz monkfish tails

200g/7oz very low-fat natural yogurt

finely grated zest and juice of 1 lime

1 tbsp dried mixed herbs

1 tbsp Worcestershire sauce

2 tsp garlic salt

1 tsp celery salt

freshly ground black pepper

16 cherry tomatoes

Fry Light for spraying

Skin and remove the thin membrane from the monkfish tails. Cut the fish into bite-sized cubes. Place in a single layer in a shallow, non-reactive dish.

Mix together the yogurt, lime zest and juice, dried herbs, Worcestershire sauce, garlic salt, celery salt and season well with freshly ground black pepper. Mix thoroughly and pour this mixture over the fish. Toss to coat evenly, cover and allow to marinate for 3–4 hours.

When ready to cook, turn the grill to medium–high. Thread the marinated fish pieces alternately with the cherry tomatoes onto eight metal skewers. Place on a foil-lined grill rack and spray with Fry Light. Grill for 6–7 minutes on each side or until cooked through and lightly coloured. Serve immediately.

GRILLED SWORDFISH WITH **ROASTED RED PEPPER GREMOLATA**

Gremolata is a delicious Mediterranean salsa or coating that goes particularly well with a meaty fish like swordfish, tuna or salmon.

serves 4 preparation time **20 minutes + marinating** cooking time **10 minutes**

4 thick swordfish steaks (you could use
   tuna or salmon if preferred)
juice of 2 lemons
2 tsp paprika
2 tbsp soy sauce
salt and freshly ground black pepper
for the gremolata
2 large red peppers
a large bunch of flat-leaf parsley, finely
   chopped

¹/₂ small red onion, peeled and finely
   chopped
finely grated zest and juice of 1 lemon
2 garlic cloves, peeled and finely
   grated
to garnish
lemon wedges

Place the swordfish steaks in a shallow, non-reactive dish in a single layer. Mix together the lemon juice, paprika and soy sauce and season well. Spoon this over the steaks, cover and leave to marinate for 15–20 minutes.

Meanwhile, make the gremolata. Place the peppers under a hot grill, turning often until blackened and blistered. Remove from the grill and place in a plastic bag for 10 minutes. When cool enough to handle, carefully peel off the skin, saving any juices from the peppers in a bowl. Deseed and finely chop the peppers and add to the bowl with the parsley, red onion, lemon zest and juice and garlic. Season well and toss to combine.

Heat a non-stick ridged griddle pan until very hot. Add the fish and cook on each side for 3–4 minutes or until just cooked through. Serve immediately with the gremolata spooned over and garnish with lemon wedges.

Original: **Free**

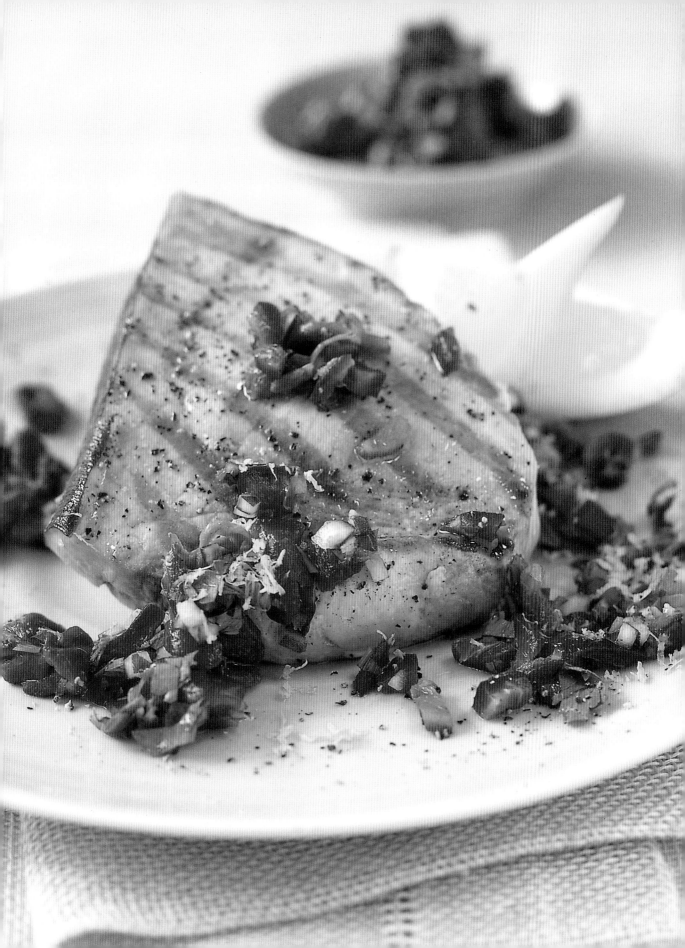

PLAICE TURBANS, MEDITERRANEAN-STYLE

This is a light and very attractive-looking dish that combines fillets of fresh plaice with a rich, slightly spicy tomato sauce – well worth the time it takes to make the 'turbans'.

serves 4   preparation time **20 minutes**   cooking time **30 minutes**

6 spring onions, trimmed and finely chopped

2 garlic cloves, peeled and crushed

1 red pepper, deseeded and finely diced

1 x 400g/14oz can chopped tomatoes

2 tbsp balsamic vinegar

2 tbsp artificial sweetener

2 tsp dried herbs de Provence

salt and freshly ground black pepper

4 plaice fillets, skinned

Fry Light for spraying

to garnish

chopped fresh basil

Preheat the oven to 190°C/Gas 5. Place the spring onions in a non-stick frying pan with the garlic, pepper, tomatoes, balsamic vinegar, sweetener and dried herbs. Bring to the boil and cook over a medium heat for 12–15 minutes, stirring often, until the mixture has reduced and thickened. Season.

Place the fish fillets on a clean work surface and cut each one in half, lengthways. Carefully spread half the tomato mixture along the surface of the fish. Roll up from the tail end to form a 'turban' and secure with a cocktail stick. Repeat with the remaining fillets.

Spray a shallow ovenproof dish with Fry Light and place the rolled 'turbans' of fish in a single layer to fit snugly. Cover lightly with foil and bake in the oven for 10–12 minutes or until the fish is cooked through.

To serve, carefully remove the fish from the ovenproof dish and place onto warmed plates. Spoon over the remaining tomato sauce, garnish with basil and serve immediately.

Original: Free

FRIED CITRUS MACKEREL FILLETS

In this recipe, the mackerel is lightly fried and then left to cool, marinating in lemon juice, which finishes the 'cooking' – a classic way to serve this rich, tasty fish.

serves 4   preparation time **15 minutes + marinating**   cooking time **6 minutes**

4 large mackerel fillets

salt and freshly ground black pepper

Fry Light for spraying

500ml/18fl oz lemon juice

2 tbsp artificial sweetener

4 shallots, peeled and very thinly sliced

1 carrot, peeled and very finely diced

1 red pepper, deseeded and very finely diced

4 tbsp finely chopped flat-leaf parsley

Season the mackerel fillets well. Spray a large non-stick frying pan with Fry Light and place over a high heat. Cook the fish, flesh side down, for 1 minute, then turn over and sear the other side for a minute. Transfer the fish, carefully, to a shallow, non-reactive dish to fit snugly in a single layer.

Wipe out the frying pan with kitchen paper and add the lemon juice, sweetener, shallots, carrot and red pepper. Bring to the boil, reduce the heat and simmer for 2 minutes. Pour this mixture over the fish. Allow to cool, cover tightly with cling film and chill and marinate in the fridge for 24 hours.

Remove the fish from the marinade and serve sprinkled with parsley. Accompany with steamed vegetables or a crisp green salad.

SPICY GRILLED SARDINES WITH MINT AND CUCUMBER RAITA

Sardines are an oily fish that contain essential fatty acids – an important part of a healthy diet. Here they are teamed with eastern spices and a cooling raita; imagine you've just caught and cooked them on the beach!

serves 4 preparation time **15 minutes + chilling** cooking time **10 minutes**

for the raita

1 cucumber, finely diced

2 tomatoes, finely diced

1 small red onion, peeled and finely diced

6 tbsp chopped mint leaves

200g/7oz very low-fat natural yogurt

salt and freshly ground black pepper

for the sardines

12 sardines, gutted and cleaned

juice of 2 lemons

1 tsp hot chilli powder

1 tsp ground cumin

1 tsp ground coriander

Fry Light for spraying

to serve

mint sprigs

Make the raita by putting all the ingredients into a bowl. Mix well, season, cover and chill until ready to use.

Place the sardines in a shallow, non-reactive dish, in a single layer. Mix together the lemon juice, chilli powder, ground cumin and ground coriander. Season well with salt and spoon this mixture over the sardines. Cover and chill for 15–20 minutes.

When ready to cook, preheat the grill to hot. Place the sardines in a single layer on a large grill rack, spray with Fry Light and cook under the grill for 4–5 minutes on each side or until cooked through and lightly charred. Serve immediately garnished with mint sprigs and with the mint and cucumber raita in a bowl alongside.

Original: Free

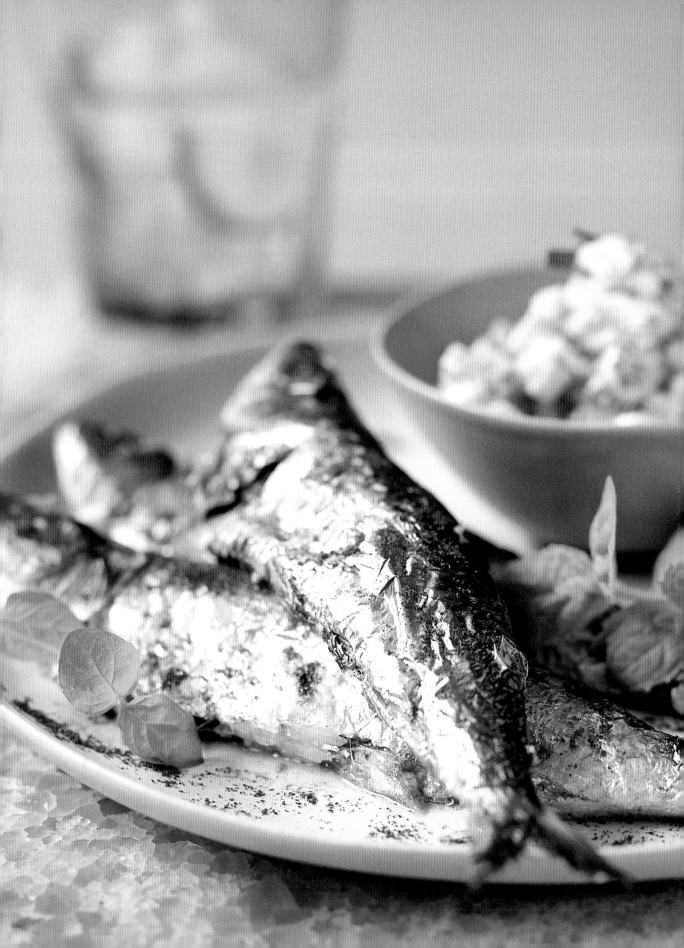

POACHED HALIBUT IN CUCUMBER SAUCE

Halibut is a delicately flavoured fish that lends itself very well to a fresh, savoury cucumber sauce.

serves 4 preparation time **15 minutes** cooking time **15 minutes**

4 halibut fillets (approximately
    250g/9oz each), skinned
for the sauce
150g/5oz cucumber, very finely diced
1 small onion, peeled and finely diced
600ml/1 pint chicken stock made from
    Bovril

4 tbsp chopped fresh dill
2 tbsp finely chopped chives
1 green chilli, deseeded and very finely
    chopped
salt and freshly ground black pepper
to garnish
lime wedges

Preheat the oven to 150°C/Gas 2. Place the fish in a large non-stick saucepan, cover with water and poach for 6–8 minutes or until cooked through. Carefully transfer to a non-stick baking sheet and keep warm in the oven.

Make the sauce by placing the cucumber, onion and stock in a small saucepan. Bring to the boil, reduce the heat and cook gently for 5–6 minutes. Add the chopped herbs and green chilli, season well and transfer to a food processor. Blend until smooth.

To serve, place the poached fish onto warmed plates and spoon the sauce over and around them. Serve garnished with wedges of lime.

SALMON FILLET PROVENÇALE

Roasted Mediterranean vegetables add colour and flavour to a filling dish of pan-fried salmon that's quick to put together, yet looks very impressive.

serves 4   preparation time **20 minutes**   cooking time **30 minutes**

1 yellow pepper, deseeded and cut into 2cm/³/₄in pieces

1 red pepper, deseeded and cut into 2cm/³/₄in pieces

1 courgette, cut into 2cm/³/₄in pieces

1 aubergine, cut into 2cm/³/₄in pieces

1 red onion, peeled and roughly diced

1 tbsp garlic salt

Fry Light for spraying

2 tbsp chopped rosemary leaves

salt and freshly ground black pepper

4 thick salmon fillets, skinned

to serve

lemon wedges

Preheat the oven to 220°C/Gas 7. Place the peppers, courgette, aubergine and onion in a single layer on a large non-stick baking sheet or roasting tin. Sprinkle over the garlic salt, spray with Fry Light and sprinkle over the rosemary. Season well and place in the oven and cook for 15–20 minutes or until the vegetables are tender and slightly charred at the edges.

Meanwhile, spray the salmon with Fry Light and season well. Heat a large non-stick griddle pan over a high heat and then cook the salmon for about 3–4 minutes on each side or until cooked through. Transfer onto warmed serving plates. Spoon over the roasted vegetables and serve with wedges of lemon to squeeze over.

PARCHMENT FISH PARCELS

Cooking fish in a parcel, or 'en papillote', is a great way to keep in all the juices and flavours – there's no need to add fat, and the aroma when you open the parcel at the table is wonderful.

serves 4 preparation time **20 minutes** cooking time **25 minutes**

8 spring onions, trimmed and finely shredded

1 carrot, peeled and finely julienned

1 red pepper, deseeded and finely sliced

50g/2oz mangetout, very thinly sliced

3 tbsp soy sauce

juice of 2 lemons

1 garlic clove, peeled and finely grated

1 tsp finely grated ginger

4 thick salmon fillets, skinned

salt and freshly ground black pepper

Preheat the oven to 200°C/Gas 6. Cut four squares of baking parchment paper, large enough to comfortably wrap each piece of fish.

In a large bowl, mix together the spring onions, carrot, red pepper, mangetout, soy sauce, lemon juice, garlic and ginger. Divide this mixture between the four squares of baking parchment and top each one with a salmon fillet. Season well and fold the paper over the fish to form a parcel, with the edges firmly sealed. Place the parcels on a baking sheet and place in the oven for 20–25 minutes or until the fish is just cooked through.

Remove from the oven and place the parcels onto warmed serving plates. Unwrap the parcels at the table and eat immediately.

Original: Free

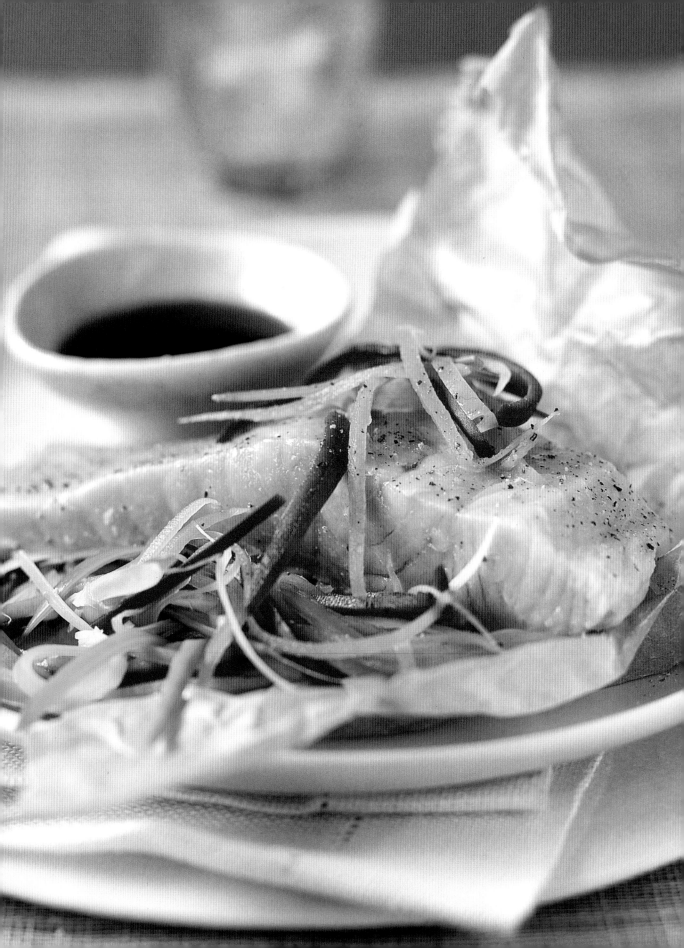

VEGETABLES

GREEN BEANS WITH PUY LENTILS

Lentils have a nutty, earthy taste that's very moreish. Here they are cooked with spices, tomatoes and fresh, crunchy green beans for a burst of flavour and texture.

serves 4 preparation time **30 minutes** cooking time **10 minutes**

100g/4oz puy lentils, rinsed and
  drained
400g/14oz fresh green beans, trimmed
  and halved
Fry Light for spraying
1 onion, peeled and finely chopped
1 garlic clove, peeled and finely sliced
1 tsp finely grated ginger

2 tsp cumin seeds
1 tsp ground coriander
1 red chilli, deseeded and finely sliced
3 tomatoes, roughly chopped
large handful of coriander and mint,
  chopped
salt and freshly ground black pepper

Place the lentils in a large saucepan and cover liberally with cold water. Bring to the boil and cook over a medium heat for 25–30 minutes or until tender. Drain and set aside.

While the lentils are cooking, boil the green beans for 8–10 minutes until just tender, drain and set aside.

Spray a large non-stick frying pan with Fry Light and place over a medium heat. Add the onion, garlic, ginger, cumin seeds, ground coriander and red chilli. Stir-fry for 2–3 minutes and then add 100ml/3$\frac{1}{2}$fl oz water and continue to stir and cook for 3–4 minutes. Add the lentils, beans and tomatoes and cook over a high heat for 2–3 minutes. Stir in the chopped herbs, season and serve immediately.

Green: **Free**

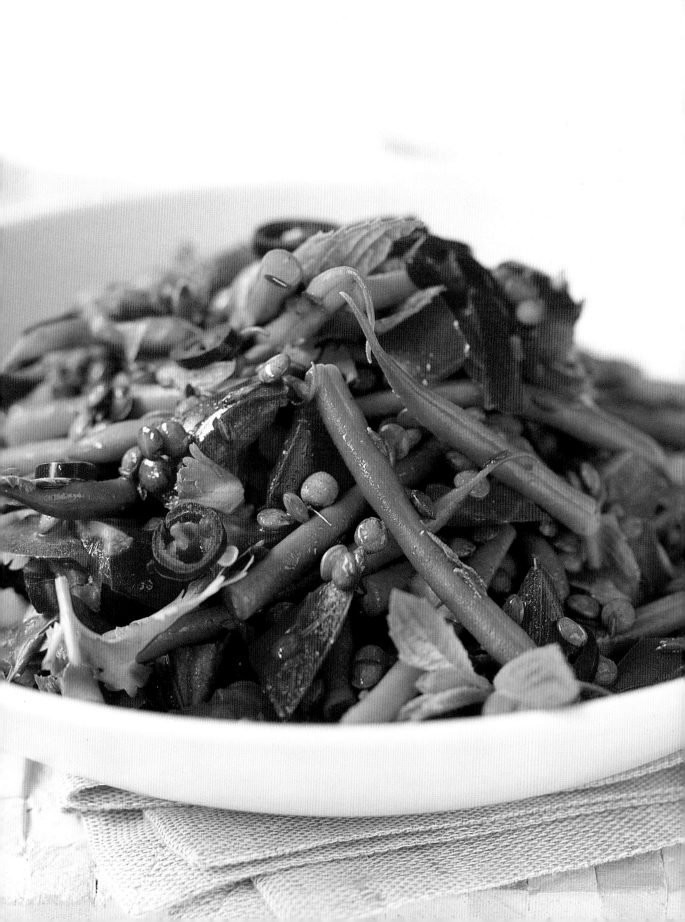

TEX MEX CHILLI

Chilli is always a favourite and this version has extra vegetables for filling power. It tastes great on a pile of fluffy boiled rice.

serves 4 preparation time **20 minutes** cooking time **45 minutes**

Fry Light for spraying

1 large onion, peeled and finely chopped

2 garlic cloves, peeled and crushed

2 tsp ground cumin

1 tsp ground cinnamon

1 red chilli, deseeded and finely chopped

2 large carrots, peeled and cut into small dice

1 red pepper, deseeded and finely chopped

2 courgettes, cut into small dice

8 ripe plum tomatoes

500ml/18fl oz passata

1 tbsp soy sauce

1 tsp Tabasco sauce

1 tbsp artificial sweetener

1 x 400g/14oz can red kidney beans

8 tbsp finely chopped fresh coriander

salt and freshly ground black pepper

Spray a large non-stick saucepan with Fry Light. Place over a medium heat and add the onion. Stir and cook for 4–5 minutes or until softened then add the garlic. Stir and fry for 2–3 minutes before adding the cumin, cinnamon, chilli, carrots, red pepper and courgettes. Stir and cook for 3–4 minutes.

Roughly chop the tomatoes and add to the saucepan with the passata, soy sauce, Tabasco sauce and sweetener. Bring to the boil, reduce the heat, cover and cook gently for 30 minutes, stirring occasionally.

Rinse and drain the beans and add to the saucepan. Heat through for 3–4 minutes then remove from the heat and stir in the chopped coriander and seasoning. Serve ladled into warmed bowls.

Green: **Free**

VEGETABLE MADRAS CURRY

This is the perfect 'storecupboard curry' – it's made with ingredients that are nearly always on hand in the larder or the freezer, and it makes a great family supper at any time of year.

serves 4   preparation time **20 minutes**   cooking time **45 minutes**

Fry Light for spraying

700g/1lb 9oz potatoes, peeled and cut into bite-sized cubes

2 onions, peeled and roughly chopped

3 garlic cloves, peeled and crushed

1 tbsp Madras curry powder

1 tsp finely grated ginger

300g/11oz cauliflower florets

4 ripe plum tomatoes, chopped

100g/4oz frozen peas

4 tbsp chopped fresh coriander

350ml/12fl oz chicken stock made from Bovril

1 tbsp artificial sweetener

salt

150g/5oz very low-fat natural yogurt

Spray a large non-stick saucepan with Fry Light. Add the potatoes, onions and garlic and cook over a medium heat for 3–4 minutes. Add the curry powder and ginger and stir and cook for 1 minute.

Add the cauliflower, tomatoes, frozen peas, coriander, stock and sweetener. Bring to the boil, reduce the heat, cover and cook gently for 30–35 minutes, stirring often until the vegetables are tender. Remove from the heat, season well and stir in the yogurt just before serving.

BARLEY AND BUTTERNUT SQUASH HOT POT

Butternut squash is widely on sale in supermarkets and is tasty and easy to cook with. Here it makes a savoury, satisfying stew with a silky texture that comes from the pearl barley.

serves 4   preparation time **15 minutes**   cooking time **1 hour 20 minutes**

50g/2oz pearl barley

2 carrots, peeled and cut into thick
   slices

2 garlic cloves, peeled and crushed

1 bouquet garni

1 litre/1³/₄ pints chicken stock made
   from Bovril

800g/1lb 12oz butternut squash,
   peeled, deseeded and flesh cut into
   bite-sized pieces

salt and freshly ground black pepper

to garnish

chopped thyme leaves

Place the barley in a large saucepan, cover with water and bring to the boil. Cook for 45 minutes or until tender. Drain and return to the saucepan with the carrots, garlic, bouquet garni and stock. Bring to the boil, cover, reduce the heat to medium and simmer gently for 15–20 minutes.

Add the butternut squash and continue to cook gently for 10–15 minutes. Season well, discard the bouquet garni and serve immediately, garnished with chopped thyme leaves.

Green: **Free**

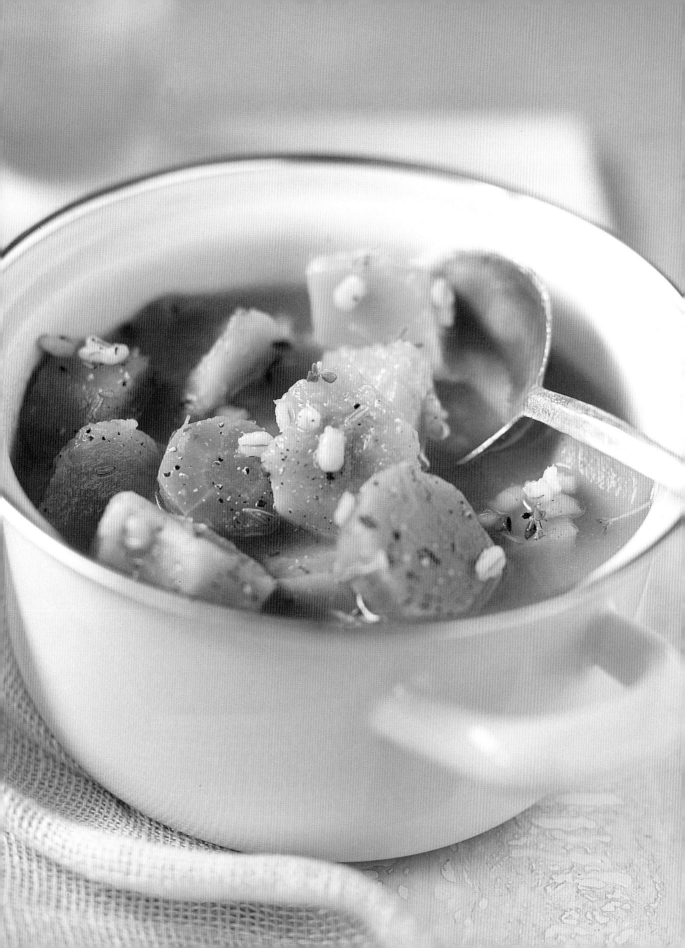

POTATO-TOPPED BEAN PIE

This is a super-healthy, super-filling supper dish that's packed full of vitamins and fibre – comfort food that tastes so good everyone will want seconds!

serves 4 preparation time **20 minutes** cooking time **1 hour**

Fry Light for spraying

2 garlic cloves, peeled and crushed

2 leeks, trimmed and thinly sliced

250g/9oz parsnips, peeled and diced

2 carrots, peeled and diced

2 sticks of celery, diced

2 tsp dried oregano

1 x 400g/14oz can mixed beans in
  chilli sauce

150g/5oz passata with garlic and
  herbs

1 tbsp artificial sweetener

150ml/5fl oz chicken stock made
  from Bovril

salt and freshly ground black pepper

for the topping

1.5kg/3lb 6oz potatotes (Desirée or
  Maris Piper)

1 egg, beaten

salt and freshly ground black pepper

Preheat the oven to 200°C/Gas 6. Spray a large non-stick frying pan with Fry Light. Add the garlic and cook over a medium heat for 1 minute. Stir in the leeks, parsnips, carrots, celery and oregano. Stir and cook for 3–4 minutes.

Add the beans, passata, sweetener, stock and seasoning and bring to the boil. Reduce the heat, cover and simmer gently for 20 minutes.

Meanwhile, boil the potatoes in a large saucepan of lightly salted water until tender. Then drain, return to the pan and mash until fairly smooth. Cool and add the egg, season and stir to mix well. Set aside.

Spoon the bean and vegetable mixture into an ovenproof dish. Spread the potato mixture carefully over to cover and place in the oven and bake for 25–30 minutes until the top is golden brown and bubbling. Serve immediately.

Green: **Free**

CHUNKY ROASTED BROCCOLI WITH GARLIC AND HERBS

A very fresh and colourful way of cooking broccoli and peppers, this is a versatile dish that would be a filling lunch or a delicious accompaniment to rice or pasta on a Green day, or meat or fish on Original days.

serves 4 preparation time **15 minutes** cooking time **20 minutes**

1kg/2lb 4oz broccoli

Fry Light for spraying

3 red peppers, deseeded and cut into thick strips

6 garlic cloves, peeled and thinly sliced

1 red chilli, deseeded and thinly sliced

salt and freshly ground black pepper to garnish

a handful of flat-leaf parsley and basil leaves

Cut the broccoli into chunky florets. Bring a large saucepan of lightly salted water to the boil. Add the broccoli and boil for 3–4 minutes. Drain and refresh under cold water. Drain and set aside.

Preheat the oven to 220°C/Gas 7. Line a large baking sheet with non-stick baking parchment and spray with Fry Light. Place the pepper strips on the prepared baking sheet with the broccoli in a single layer.

Scatter the garlic and chilli over the vegetables. Season well and spray the vegetables with Fry Light. Place in the oven and roast for 15–20 minutes. Remove from the oven and transfer to a serving dish with any of the juices. Scatter over the chopped herbs and serve warm or at room temperature.

SPINACH AND SWEET POTATO CURRY

This is a fresh-tasting curry that would be a very satisfying supper served with a pile of steamed Basmati rice, or as part of a delicious Indian buffet.

serves 4   preparation time **15 minutes**   cooking time **18 minutes**

300ml/½ pint vegetable stock or
  chicken stock made from Bovril
750g/1lb 10oz sweet potatoes, peeled
  and cut into bite-sized wedges
1 onion, peeled, halved and thinly
  sliced

225g/8oz fresh baby spinach leaves
2 garlic cloves, peeled and thinly sliced
1 red chilli, deseeded and thinly sliced
1 tbsp medium or hot curry powder
4 ripe plum tomatoes, chopped
salt and freshly ground black pepper

Place the stock in a large saucepan and add the sweet potatoes and onions. Bring to the boil, reduce the heat, cover and gently cook for 4–5 minutes.

Add the spinach, garlic, chilli, curry powder and tomatoes to the saucepan, stir well and cook over a medium heat for 10 minutes or until the spinach has just wilted and the sweet potatoes are tender. Season well and serve hot.

Green: **Free**

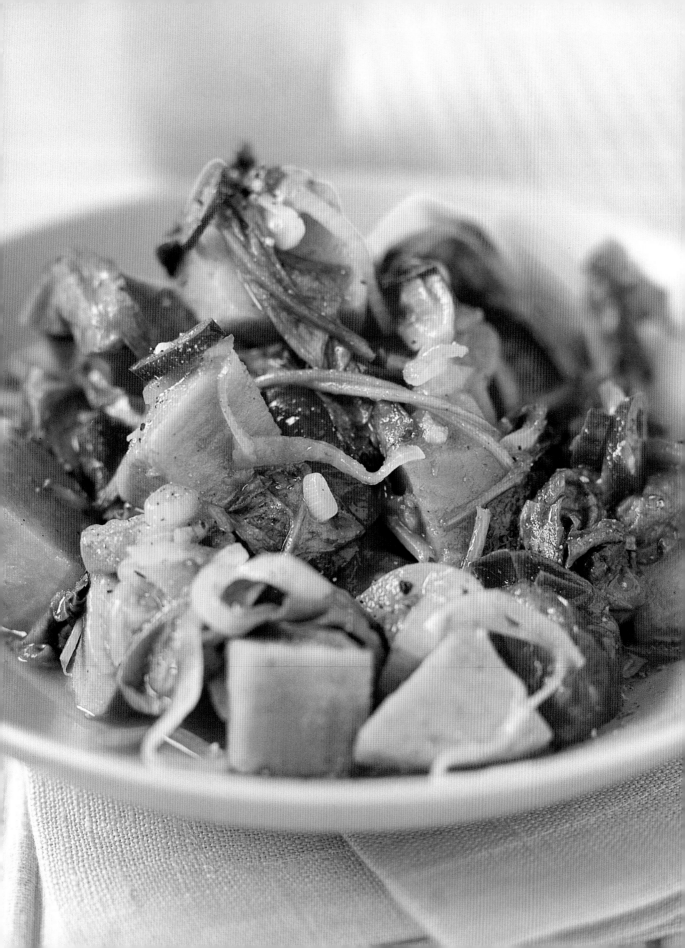

ITALIAN-STYLE COURGETTES

Making courgettes into a very special supper dish or vegetable side-dish is easy with this all-in-one-pan recipe. The creamy onion-flavoured sauce would also work well with pasta.

serves 4 preparation time **15 minutes** cooking time **12 minutes**

Fry Light for spraying

800g/1lb 12oz large courgettes, cut into 1cm/½in slices

1 red onion, peeled, halved and thinly sliced

150ml/5fl oz chicken stock made from Bovril

4 tbsp chopped flat-leaf parsley

2 tbsp finely chopped mint leaves

200g/7oz very low-fat natural fromage frais

salt and freshly ground black pepper

Spray a large non-stick saucepan with Fry Light and place over a medium heat. Add the courgette and the onion and stir-fry for 2–3 minutes.

Pour in the stock, cover and cook on a gentle heat for 6–8 minutes, stirring occasionally or until the courgettes are just tender.

Add the parsley and mint, remove from the heat and stir in the fromage frais. Season well and serve immediately.

Green/Original: **Free**

ROOT VEGETABLE, CABBAGE AND HERB MASH

Give bubble and squeak an exotic twist by using celeriac and sweet potato, and mixing up the mash with a tangy, creamy dressing. You could use this versatile dish as a topping for vegetable or Quorn cottage pie – or for a hearty winter brunch.

serves 4 preparation time **20 minutes** cooking time **35 minutes**

500g/1lb 2oz sweet potato, peeled and roughly chopped

500g/1lb 2oz celeriac, peeled and roughly chopped

Fry Light for spraying

4 spring onions, trimmed and thinly sliced

300g/11oz green cabbage, thinly shredded

6 tbsp very low-fat natural yogurt

4 tbsp very low-fat natural fromage frais

1 tsp mustard powder

4 tbsp finely chopped flat-leaf parsley

salt and freshly ground black pepper

Bring a large pan of lightly salted water to the boil and add the chopped vegetables. Boil for 15–20 minutes or until tender, drain and return to the pan and, using a potato masher, mash roughly. Set aside and keep warm.

Spray a large non-stick wok or frying pan with Fry Light and place over a high heat. Add the spring onions and cabbage to the pan and stir and cook for 3–4 minutes. Add 5–6 tablespoons of water, reduce the heat to low, cover tightly and allow to cook gently for 3–4 minutes, stirring occasionally.

Stir the cabbage mixture into the root vegetable mash and stir to combine.

Beat together the yogurt and fromage frais. Mix the mustard with a tablespoon of water and add to the yogurt mixture. Stir this into the mash and combine well. Scatter over the chopped herbs, season well and serve.

CABBAGE AND CARROT STIR-FRY

Cooking vegetables lightly preserves their nutrients so this stir-fry is very healthy as well as quick and tasty. It would go well with noodles on a Green day or grilled meat on an Original day.

serves 4   preparation time **20 minutes**   cooking time **10 minutes**

3 carrots, peeled

2 garlic cloves, peeled and thinly sliced

1 red onion, peeled and thinly sliced

200g/7oz sweetheart cabbage, finely
  shredded

Fry Light for spraying

1 tsp ground ginger

2 tsp ground Cajun spice

juice of 1 lemon

salt and freshly ground black pepper

Using a mandolin or vegetable shredder, thinly slice the carrots to get thin julienne strips. Prepare the rest of the vegetables.

Spray a large non-stick wok with Fry Light and place over a high heat. Add the garlic and onion and stir-fry for 2–3 minutes.

Add the carrots, cabbage, ginger, Cajun spice and stir-fry for 5–6 minutes. Add the lemon juice, remove from the heat, season well and serve immediately.

Green/Original **Free**

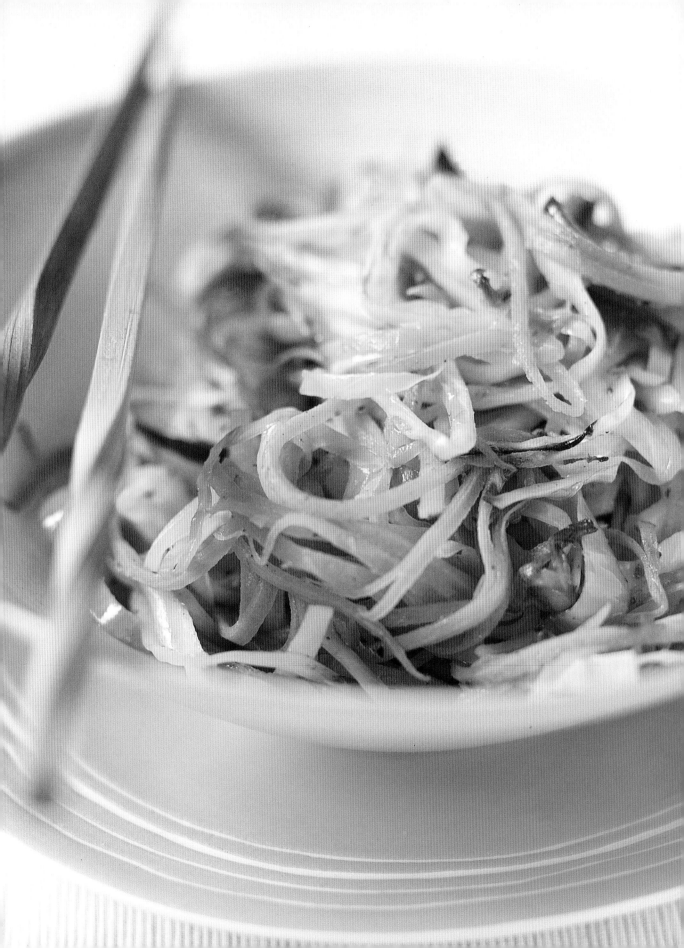

CHICKPEA AND TOMATO CASSEROLE

Potatoes and chickpeas make this colourful stew into a particularly satisfying meal that's easily whipped up using storecupboard ingredients and a few fresh vegetables.

serves 4 preparation time **15 minutes** cooking time **30 minutes**

Fry Light for spraying

1 red onion, finely sliced

2 garlic cloves, peeled and crushed

200g/7oz baby new potatoes, halved

1 tsp ground cumin

1 red pepper, deseeded and roughly
  diced

1 courgette, roughly chopped

1 x 400g/14oz can chopped tomatoes

1 x 400g/14oz can chickpeas, rinsed
  and drained

1 tbsp Worcestershire sauce

4 tbsp chopped parsley

salt and freshly ground black pepper

Spray a large non-stick frying pan with Fry Light and place over a medium heat. Add the onion, garlic and potatoes and stir and cook for 3–4 minutes.

Stir in the cumin, pepper and courgette and continue to stir and cook for 3–4 minutes.

Stir in the chopped tomatoes, chickpeas and Worcestershire sauce. Bring to the boil, cover and simmer gently for 15–20 minutes or until the vegetables are tender. Stir in the parsley and season well before serving.

Green: **Free**

BABY ROASTED POTATOES WITH FENNEL AND LEMON THYME

Everyone loves roast potatoes and these have the added fragrance and crunch of fennel seeds, garlic salt and lemon thyme – perfect served with fish.

serves 4   preparation time **15 minutes**   cooking time **35 minutes**

1.5kg/3lb 6oz baby new potatoes

Fry Light for spraying

2 tsp garlic salt

2 tbsp fennel seeds

4–5 sprigs of lemon thyme

sea salt and freshly ground black pepper

Preheat the oven to 220°C/Gas 7. Scrub the potatoes and place in a large pan of lightly salted boiling water and cook for 4–5 minutes. Drain thoroughly.

Line a large baking sheet with non-stick baking parchment. Place the potatoes on it in a single layer. Spray with Fry Light. Sprinkle over the garlic salt.

Crush the fennel seeds in a pestle and mortar or with a rolling pin, and sprinkle over the potatoes. Scatter over the sprigs of thyme and season well. Place in the oven and roast for 25–30 minutes or until crisp and golden on the outside and soft and tender within. Serve immediately or eat cold in a salad.

BRAISED RED CABBAGE WITH RED ONIONS

Anyone who doesn't like cabbage will be converted by this wonderfully tasty, warming dish that would be a brilliant accompaniment to cold roast meat or ham, especially at Christmas as it has a festive, spicy taste.

serves 4   preparation time **15 minutes**   cooking time **12 minutes**

1.5kg/3lb 6oz red cabbage

2 red onions

Fry Light for spraying

salt and freshly ground black pepper

1 tsp ground cinnamon

3 tbsp red wine vinegar

juice of 1 lemon

3 tbsp artificial sweetener

to garnish

chopped parsley

Halve the cabbage, take out the core and then very finely slice into thin shreds. Peel the onions and cut into thin slices.

Spray a large non-stick frying pan with Fry Light and place over a high heat. Add the cabbage and onion and stir-fry for 4–5 minutes until the cabbage has softened slightly. Season well and add the cinnamon, red wine vinegar and lemon juice.

Continue to stir and cook over a high heat for another 5–6 minutes or until the cabbage is just tender but still has a 'bite' to it. Stir in the sweetener and toss to mix well.

Remove from the heat and serve, garnished with chopped parsley.

Green/Original **Free**

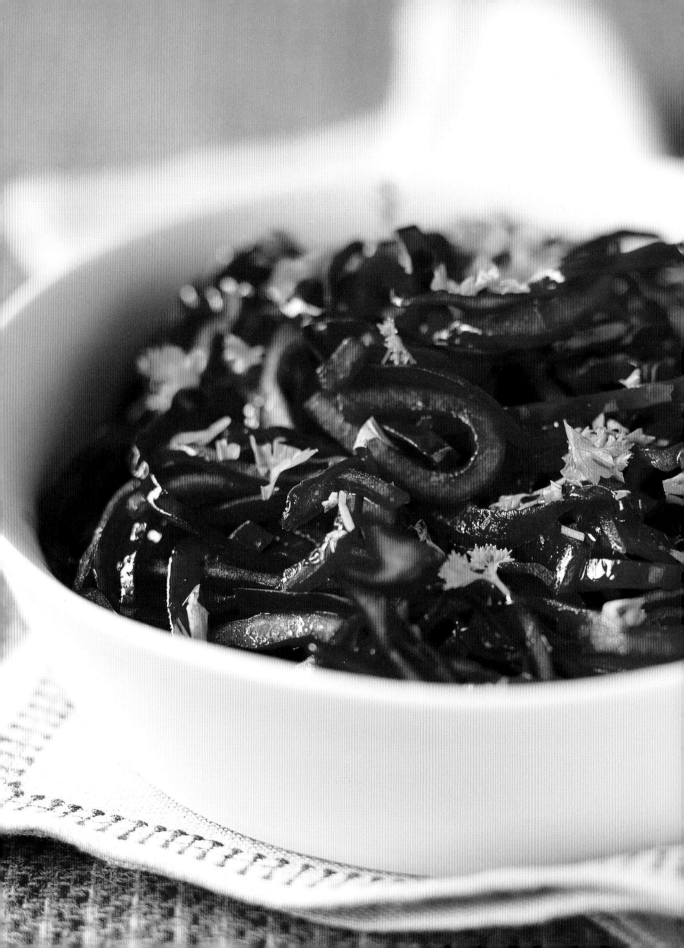

EGYPTIAN-STYLE BEAN MEDLEY

The combination of cooked beans, raw vegetables and boiled egg in a tangy dressing makes a very special savoury salad that works well in a lunchbox.

serves 4 preparation time **20 minutes + overnight soaking** cooking time **1 hour**

250g/9oz dried haricot beans

250g/9oz green beans, halved
lengthways

2 garlic cloves, peeled and crushed

4 spring onions, trimmed and very
thinly sliced

2 plum tomatoes, roughly chopped

5 tbsp roughly chopped flat-leaf parsley

salt and freshly ground black pepper

juice of 1 lemon

2 tbsp fat-free French-style salad
dressing

4 hard-boiled eggs, peeled and finely
chopped

Soak the dried haricot beans in cold water for 24 hours. Drain and then refresh under cold running water. Transfer the beans to a large saucepan and cover with cold water. Bring to the boil, reduce the heat and cook gently for 45 minutes or until the beans are tender. Drain well and transfer to a serving bowl. Keep warm.

Meanwhile, place the green beans in a saucepan of lightly salted boiling water. Boil for 5–6 minutes until just tender, drain and add to the haricot beans. Stir in the garlic, spring onions, tomatoes and parsley and season well.

Squeeze over the lemon juice and stir in the salad dressing. Toss to mix well and scatter over the chopped hard-boiled egg. Serve immediately with a crisp green salad.

PEA AND POTATO BAKE

Cooking the potatoes and peas very slowly in stock and spices ensures that the whole dish is deliciously tender and well flavoured.

serves 4   preparation time **15 minutes**   cooking time **1 hour 40 minutes**

Fry Light for spraying

700g/1lb 9oz potatoes (Desirée or
   Maris Piper), peeled and thinly sliced

2 leeks, trimmed and thinly sliced

4 plum tomatoes, thinly sliced

200g/7oz frozen peas

2 tsp chopped fresh oregano leaves

2 tsp garlic salt

1 tsp celery salt

300ml/½ pint chicken stock made
   from Bovril

freshly ground black pepper

Preheat the oven to 180°C/Gas 4. Spray a shallow ovenproof dish with Fry Light.

Layer the potatoes, leeks, tomatoes and peas in the dish, scattering the oregano leaves between each layer. Finish the top layer with potatoes. Add the garlic and celery salts to the stock and carefully pour over the potato mixture. Season well with pepper.

Cover with foil and bake in the oven for 1 hour 30 minutes. Remove the foil, and cook for 10 minutes uncovered before removing from the oven and serving.

NOODLES

PASTA

RICE

GRAINS

RUSTIC MINESTRONE

Minestrone is a meal in itself and this version is quickly put together with storecupboard ingredients, yet tastes fresh and light.

serves 4 preparation time **15 minutes** cooking time **35 minutes**

2 onions, peeled and finely chopped

2 garlic cloves, peeled and finely sliced

4 sticks of celery, cut into 1cm/½in cubes

2 large carrots, peeled and cut into 1cm/½in cubes

1 x 200g/7oz can mixed beans

Fry Light for spraying

1 x 400g/14oz can chopped tomatoes

900ml/1½ pints chicken stock made from Bovril

50g/2oz small dried pasta shapes

100g/4oz frozen peas

salt and freshly ground black pepper

4 tbsp chopped flat-leaf parsley

Prepare the vegetables and and drain and rinse the canned beans.

Spray a large saucepan with Fry Light, add the prepared vegetables and beans and stir-fry over a medium heat for 4–5 minutes. Add the tomatoes and stock and bring to the boil. Reduce the heat, cover and cook gently for 15–20 minutes, stirring occasionally.

Stir in the pasta and peas and cook for a further 6–8 minutes or until the pasta is cooked and tender. Season well, stir in the parsley and serve immediately.

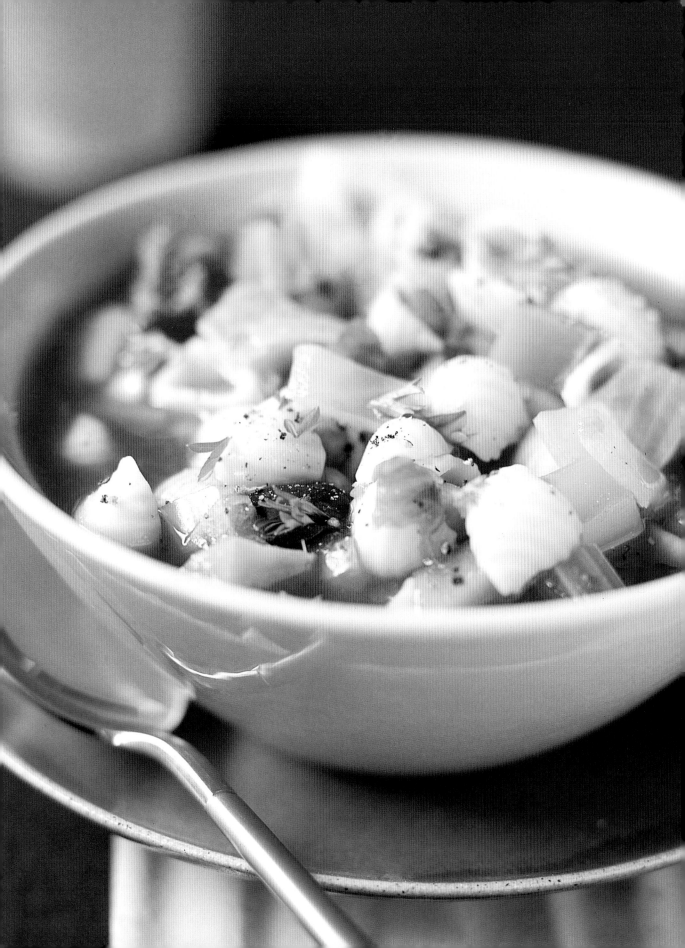

MIXED MUSHROOM NOODLE STIR-FRY

Using a variety of different mushrooms adds a depth of flavour to a crunchy, filling stir-fry with a hint of spicy warmth from ginger and soy sauce.

serves 4 preparation time **20 minutes** cooking time **10 minutes**

350g/12oz dried egg noodles

Fry Light for spraying

2.5cm/1in piece of ginger, peeled and finely julienned

2 garlic cloves, peeled and thinly sliced

6 spring onions, trimmed and cut diagonally into 3cm/1¼in pieces

200g/7oz baby corn, halved lengthways

1 red pepper, deseeded and thinly sliced

300g/11oz shiitake mushrooms, thickly sliced

200g/7oz button mushrooms, thickly sliced

150g/5oz oyster mushrooms, thickly sliced

3 tbsp dark soy sauce

freshly ground black pepper

Cook the egg noodles as on the packet instructions, drain and set aside.

Spray a large non-stick wok with Fry Light and when hot add the ginger, garlic and spring onions. Stir-fry for 1–2 minutes and then add the baby corn, pepper and mushrooms. Stir and fry over a high heat for 3–4 minutes, until the vegetables are only just tender.

Add the soy sauce with 2 tbsp water and cook for 1 minute before adding the cooked noodles. Toss to mix well and cook for 2–3 minutes, until the noodles are heated through. Season well with pepper and ladle into warmed bowls.

Green: **Free**

SINGAPORE-STYLE STIR-FRY NOODLES

Plenty of lightly cooked vegetables in this dish ensure it's as healthy as it is tasty; prepare the ingredients before you start stir-frying so that everything cooks together quickly for maximum crunch and flavour.

serves 4   preparation time **15 minutes**   cooking time **20 minutes**

2 garlic cloves, peeled and crushed

1 tsp finely grated ginger

1 red onion, peeled and chopped

60ml/2fl oz chicken stock made from Bovril

2 tbsp Worcestershire sauce

2 tbsp dark soy sauce

250g/9oz flat mushrooms, roughly chopped

2 carrots, peeled and finely julienned

1 red pepper, deseeded and thinly sliced

200g/7oz mangetout, thinly sliced

salt and freshly ground black pepper

250g/9oz beansprouts

200g/7oz dried rice noodles

to garnish

chopped coriander

sliced spring onions

Place the garlic, ginger, onion, stock, Worcestershire sauce and soy sauce in a large non-stick frying pan. Heat gently and cook over a medium–low heat for 5 minutes.

Turn the heat to high and add the mushrooms, carrots, red pepper and mangetout. Stir and cook for 4–5 minutes or until the vegetables are just tender. Season well and stir in the beansprouts and cook for 2–3 minutes.

Prepare the noodles according to the packet instructions, drain and add to the vegetable mixture in the wok. Toss to mix well, garnish with chopped coriander and sliced spring onions and serve in bowls with chopsticks.

BASIL AND TOMATO PESTO PASTA

The best of Italian cooking is simple, quickly put together and bursting with fresh flavours – just like this delicious combination of a creamy pesto-style sauce coating fine linguine pasta, with juicy ripe tomatoes.

serves 4   preparation time **15 minutes**   cooking time **12 minutes**

4 garlic cloves

1 tsp finely grated lemon zest

juice of 1 lemon

8 tbsp very finely chopped fresh basil
  leaves

200g/7oz Quark soft cheese

salt and freshly ground black pepper

350g/12oz dried linguine

8 midi vine tomatoes, halved or
  quartered

to garnish

basil leaves

Peel and finely grate the garlic to a pulp and place in a food processor with the lemon zest, lemon juice, chopped basil and Quark cheese. Season well and blend until smooth.

Cook the linguine according to the packet instructions in a large saucepan and when cooked, drain and return to the saucepan. Stir in the pesto mixture and tomatoes and toss to coat evenly.

Ladle into warmed pasta bowls or plates, garnish with basil leaves and serve immediately, accompanied by a crisp green salad.

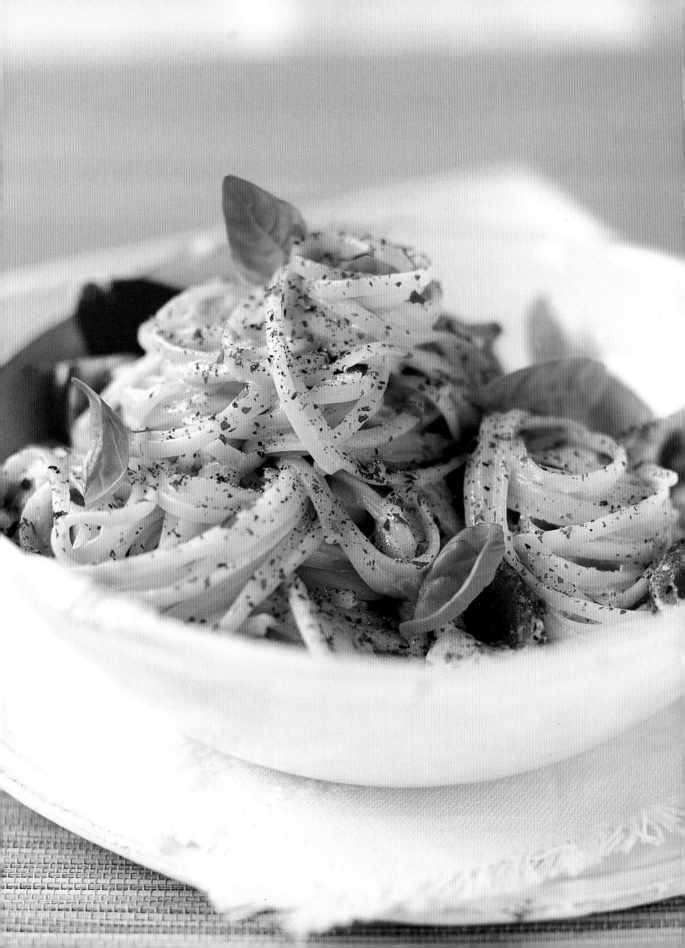

PASTA FUNGHI

Lots of fresh herbs add a wonderful fragrance and flavour to a substantial supper dish made with thick pappardelle pasta.

serves 4   preparation time **15 minutes**   cooking time **20 minutes**

350g/12oz dried pappardelle

Fry Light for spraying

1 red onion, peeled and finely diced

2 garlic cloves, peeled and finely
  chopped

400g/14oz button mushrooms, halved

500ml/18fl oz passata with herbs

1 tbsp artificial sweetener

2 tbsp chopped fresh oregano leaves

2 tbsp chopped fresh flat-leaf parsley

salt and freshly ground black pepper

50g/2oz very low-fat natural
  fromage frais

Cook the pappardelle according to the packet instructions, drain and set aside.

Spray a large non-stick frying pan with Fry Light and place over a high heat. Add the onion, garlic and mushrooms and stir-fry for 3–4 minutes.

Stir in the passata, sweetener and chopped herbs and bring to the boil. Cover, reduce the heat to low and cook gently for 15 minutes, stirring occasionally. Season well.

Just before serving, remove from the heat and stir in the fromage frais to mix well. Divide the pasta between four warmed bowls and top with the sauce.

Green: **Free**

BROCCOLI AND COURGETTE PENNE

A medley of lightly cooked green vegetables goes perfectly with tender pasta and a creamy, indulgent-tasting sauce flavoured with herbs.

serves 4 preparation time **15 minutes** cooking time **12 minutes**

350g/12oz dried penne (or any other
  short, shaped pasta)
Fry Light for spraying
2 garlic cloves, peeled and thinly sliced
6 baby leeks, trimmed and thinly sliced
250g/9oz courgettes, cut into thin
  batons
250g/9oz broccoli, separated into small
  florets

salt and freshly ground black pepper
300g/11oz very low-fat natural
  yogurt
200g/7oz Quark soft cheese
4 tbsp very finely chopped basil
2 tbsp very finely snipped chives

Cook the penne according to the packet instructions, drain and keep warm.

Spray a large non-stick wok or frying pan with Fry Light and place over a high heat. Add the garlic and prepared vegetables and stir-fry for 4–5 minutes. Add 6 tbsp of water, season well, turn the heat to low, cover and allow to cook gently for 2–3 minutes.

Meanwhile, beat the yogurt with the Quark until smooth and stir in the chopped herbs. Add the drained pasta to the vegetables in the wok or frying pan and pour in the Quark mixture. Stir to mix well and cook for 2–3 minutes until heated through. Check seasoning before serving.

CHUNKY SPAGHETTI BOLOGNESE

Everyone loves a 'spag bol' and this one is a classic recipe, except that the minced beef is replaced by Quorn, so that it is Free on a Green day – proving that it is possible to improve on perfection!

serves 4   preparation time **20 minutes**   cooking time **30 minutes**

1 onion, peeled and roughly chopped

2 large carrots, peeled and roughly diced

2 sticks of celery, roughly sliced

2 tsp dried mixed herbs

¼ tsp cayenne pepper

4 garlic cloves, peeled and crushed

150ml/5fl oz chicken stock made from Bovril

2 x 400g/14oz cans chopped tomatoes

1 tbsp artificial sweetener

350g/12oz Quorn mince

salt and freshly ground black pepper

350g/12oz dried spaghetti

to garnish

chopped flat-leaf parsley

Place the prepared vegetables in a large non-stick frying pan or wok with the dried mixed herbs, cayenne, garlic and stock. Place over a medium heat and bring to the boil. Cook for 3–4 minutes, until the vegetables begin to soften.

Stir in the chopped tomatoes, sweetener and Quorn mince. Season well, bring to the boil then cover, reduce the heat and cook gently for 20–25 minutes, stirring often, until the sauce is thick and the vegetables tender.

While the sauce is cooking, cook the pasta according to the packet instructions. Drain and keep warm.

To serve, divide the cooked spaghetti between four warmed plates and top with the chunky Bolognese sauce. Garnish with chopped parsley and serve immediately.

Green Free

CREAMY ASPARAGUS CARBONARA

Carbonara sauce is usually made with ham, but using asparagus instead is a clever way of adding colour and flavour to the dish – and would be especially good in May and June when asparagus is in season.

serves 4 preparation time **15 minutes** cooking time **10 minutes**

350g/12oz dried linguine or tagliatelle

400g/14oz asparagus tips

2 eggs

100g/4oz very low-fat natural fromage frais

1 garlic clove, peeled and crushed

6 tbsp very finely chopped flat-leaf parsley

salt and freshly ground black pepper

Fry Light for spraying

Cook the pasta according to the packet instructions, drain and keep warm.

While the pasta is cooking, blanch the asparagus tips in a pan of lightly salted boiling water for 3–4 minutes, or until just tender. Drain and set aside.

In a mixing bowl beat the eggs lightly and add the fromage frais and garlic. Whisk until well combined and then stir in the chopped parsley. Season well.

Spray a large non-stick frying pan with Fry Light and place over a medium–low heat. Add the spaghetti and asparagus to the pan and stir and cook for 2–3 minutes until hot. Pour over the 'carbonara' sauce and gently heat through for 2–3 minutes until the pasta is well coated. (Do not allow to boil or the eggs will scramble.) Remove from the heat and serve immediately.

CHILLI, CHIVE AND BEETROOT RISOTTO

The flavour of beetroot lends itself very well to a creamy risotto and garnishing it with chilli adds some spicy heat to the mix.

serves 4   preparation time **15 minutes**   cooking time **30 minutes**

Fry Light for spraying

1 red onion, peeled and finely chopped

2 garlic cloves, peeled and finely sliced

1 red chilli, deseeded and thinly sliced

500g/1lb 2oz freshly cooked peeled beetroot

1 small carrot, peeled and finely diced

2 tbsp very finely snipped chives

350g/12oz risotto rice

900ml/1½ pints chicken stock made from Bovril, boiling hot

salt and freshly ground black pepper

4 tbsp very low-fat natural yogurt

to garnish

chives

red and green chilli, deseeded and sliced (optional)

Spray a non-stick saucepan or frying pan with Fry Light. Place over a medium heat and add the onion, garlic and chilli and stir-fry for 1–2 minutes.

Chop the beetroot into small cubes and add to the pan with the carrots, chives and rice. Add the stock, a ladleful at a time, and cook over a gentle heat for 20–25 minutes, stirring continuously, until all the stock has been absorbed and the rice is creamy and *al dente*, or just firm to the bite. Add extra stock if the risotto needs it.

Season well and ladle into four warmed bowls or plates. Spoon the yogurt over each serving, garnish with chives and chillies, if desired, and serve immediately.

Green **Free**

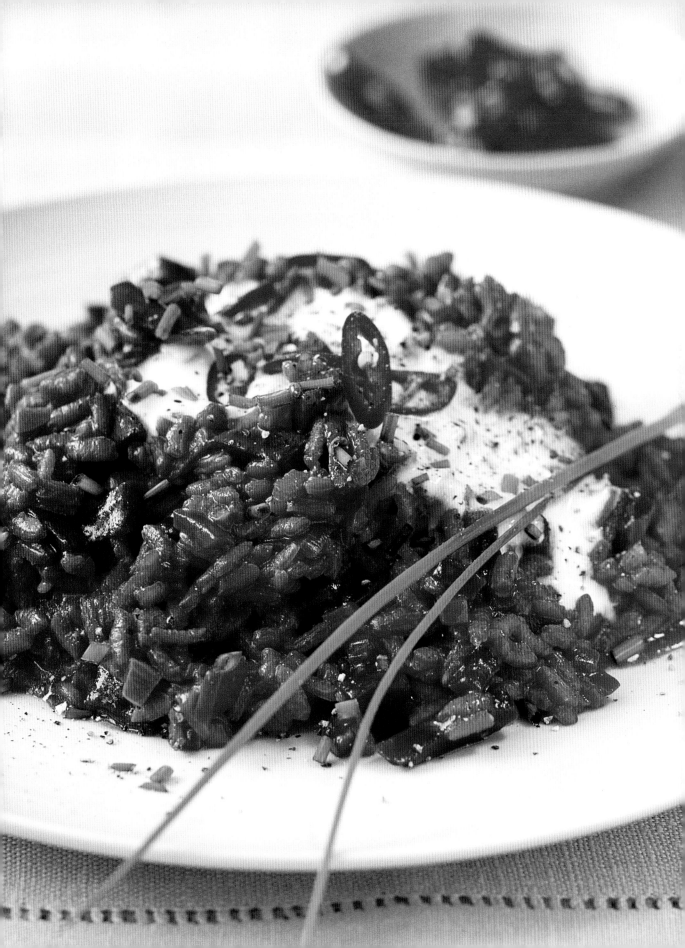

QUICK RISOTTO VERDE

Making the risotto with ready-boiled rice saves on stirring time and the addition of lots of fresh green vegetables makes this a lovely dish for a summer lunch.

serves 4 preparation time **15 minutes** cooking time **12 minutes**

- 2 leeks, trimmed and thinly sliced
- 200g/7oz mangetout, trimmed and cut into thin strips
- 200g/7oz green beans, trimmed and cut in half lengthways
- 200g/7oz frozen broad beans
- 250g/9oz frozen peas
- 500ml/18fl oz chicken stock made from Bovril
- 450g/1lb boiled Basmati rice
- 4 tbsp chopped chives
- 4 tbsp chopped dill
- salt and freshly ground black pepper

Place the leeks, mangetout, green beans, broad beans and peas into a large non-stick frying pan with the stock. Place over a high heat and bring to the boil. Reduce the heat, cover and allow to cook gently for 5–6 minutes.

Stir in the boiled rice. Bring back to the boil and stir and cook for 5–6 minutes or until all the vegetables are tender. Stir in the chopped herbs, season well and ladle into warmed bowls and serve immediately.

LENTIL AND EGG KEDGEREE

Kedgeree is traditionally made with smoked haddock; using lentils here adds a nutty taste, which combines with rice and hard-boiled egg to make an unusual and satisfying lunch or supper dish.

serves 4 preparation time **15 minutes** cooking time **30 minutes**

Fry Light for spraying

1 large onion, peeled and chopped

2 tsp mild curry powder

250g/9oz Basmati rice

50g/2oz red or yellow split lentils

1 bay leaf

1 cinnamon stick

650ml/22fl oz chicken stock made from Bovril

salt and freshly ground black pepper

8 large eggs

to garnish

chopped coriander

Spray a large non-stick frying pan with Fry Light. Place over a high heat and add the onion. Stir-fry for 2–3 minutes and then add the curry powder, rice, lentils, bay leaf and cinnamon stick. Stir and fry for 1–2 minutes.

Pour in the stock, season well and bring to the boil. Cover tightly, reduce the heat and allow to cook gently for about 15 minutes. Remove from the heat and let stand, undisturbed, for 10–12 minutes.

While the rice is standing, boil the eggs to your liking. Shell and halve them and set aside. Remove the lid from the rice, fluff up the grains with a fork and spoon into four warmed bowls or plates. Top each serving with four egg halves, sprinkle over the chopped coriander and serve immediately.

FRAGRANT SPICED VEGETABLE RICE

Spicy rice with colourful vegetables is a substantial and moreish dish either on its own or with other Green day Indian dishes, such as spiced potatoes.

serves 4   preparation time **10 minutes**   cooking time **30 minutes + standing time**

Fry Light for spraying

1 large onion, peeled, halved and
    thinly sliced

2 carrots, peeled and diced

1 courgette, trimmed and diced

60ml/2fl oz chicken stock made
    from Bovril

2 tsp ground coriander

2 tsp cumin seeds

1 tsp ground cumin

1/4 tsp crushed cardamom seeds

2 cloves

1 large cinnamon stick

1/2 tsp ground turmeric

250g/9oz Basmati rice

salt and freshly ground black pepper

Spray a large, non-stick frying pan with Fry Light. Place over a medium heat and add the onions, carrots and courgette. Stir and cook for 4–5 minutes and then add the stock and cook for a further 4–5 minutes until most of the stock has been absorbed.

Stir in the spices. Stir and cook for 1–2 minutes before stirring in the rice. Stir for a further 1–2 minutes and then pour in 600ml/1 pint water. Season well. Bring to the boil, cover tightly, reduce the heat and cook on a low heat for 12–15 minutes.

Remove from the heat and let sit undisturbed for 10–12 minutes before removing the cover. Fluff up the grains with a fork and serve immediately.

Green Free

VEGETABLE PAELLA

Saffron and smoked paprika are the traditional flavourings for paella; in this version, the chicken and seafood are replaced by colourful vegetables.

serves 4 preparation time **30 minutes** cooking time **20 minutes**

250g/9oz brown Basmati rice (or brown long grain)

300g/11oz runner beans, trimmed and cut diagonally into 2.5cm/1in pieces

1 large carrot, peeled and diced

1 head of broccoli, cut into florets

Fry Light for spraying

1 large onion, peeled and chopped

2 garlic cloves, peeled and finely chopped

a pinch of saffron threads

1 tsp sweet smoked paprika

200ml/7fl oz chicken stock made from Bovril

200g/7oz frozen peas

salt and freshly ground black pepper

2 tbsp chopped flat-leaf parsley

Cook the rice according to the packet instructions, drain and set aside.

Bring a large saucepan of lightly salted water to the boil and add the runner beans, carrot and broccoli. Boil for 8–10 minutes or until tender. Drain and set aside.

Spray a large non-stick frying pan with Fry Light and place over a medium heat. Add the onion, garlic, saffron, paprika, stock and peas, and bring to the boil. Reduce the heat and cook gently for 4–5 minutes or until the onion has softened.

Add the drained rice and vegetables to the pan, stir to mix well, cover and cook gently for 3–4 minutes. Season well, stir in the chopped parsley and serve immediately.

COUSCOUS WITH STEWED VEGETABLES

Couscous served with a spicy mix of vegetables is a classic Moroccan dish; the vegetables are very tender and the contrast of taste and texture with the soft, grainy couscous is simple and delicious.

serves 4   preparation time **20 minutes**   cooking time **40 minutes**

300g/11oz couscous

Fry Light for spraying

1 onion, peeled and finely chopped

1 tsp ground cinnamon

1 tsp ground ginger

2 tsp ground cumin

2 large carrots, peeled and cut into bite-sized pieces

1 courgette, cut into bite-sized pieces

1 medium aubergine, cut into bite-sized pieces

100g/4oz okra, trimmed

1 red pepper, deseeded and cut into bite-sized pieces

700ml/24fl oz chicken stock made from Bovril

1 x 400g/14oz can chopped tomatoes

1 tbsp artificial sweetener

salt and freshly ground black pepper

to garnish

chopped mint leaves

Prepare the couscous according to the packet instructions and keep warm.

Spray a large non-stick saucepan with Fry Light and place over a medium heat. Add the onion and the ground spices and stir-fry for 2–3 minutes.

Add the vegetables and stir-fry for 2–3 minutes. Pour in the stock, tomatoes and sweetener and bring to the boil. Cover tightly, reduce the heat to medium–low and cook gently for 20–25 minutes, stirring occasionally until the vegetables are tender. Season well.

To serve, spoon the prepared couscous into large warmed bowls and spoon over the vegetable mixture. Garnish with the mint leaves and serve immediately.

Green: **Free**

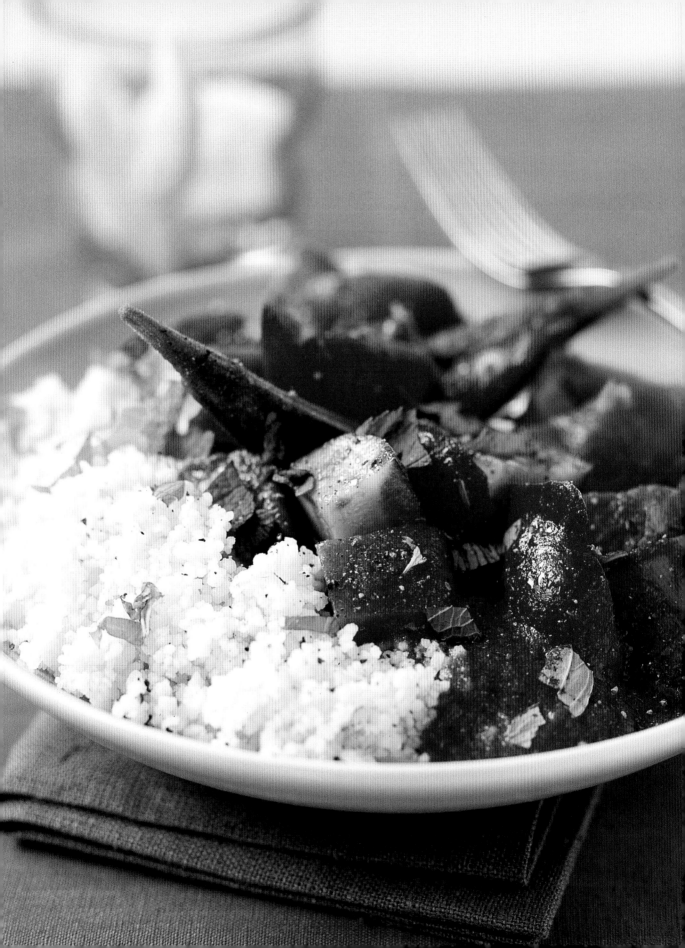

TABBOULEH

Tabbouleh is a great dish for lunchboxes as it travels well and the flavour develops when it's left to stand. Made with bulgar wheat, it's a no-cook salad that's packed with fresh, zingy flavours.

serves 4 preparation time **20 minutes + standing time**

100g/4oz bulgar wheat

750g/1lb 10oz ripe plum tomatoes

6 spring onions

2 large bunches flat-leaf parsley

50g/2oz mint leaves

juice of 3 lemons

60ml/2fl oz chicken stock made from
    Bovril

1/2 tsp ground allspice

salt and freshly ground black pepper

to serve

small cos or little gem lettuce leaves

Soak the bulgar wheat for 15–20 minutes in a large bowl of cold water until soft and swollen. Check the grains to see if tender, then drain thoroughly, pressing out any excess liquid.

Transfer the soaked bulgar wheat to a large, shallow, non-reactive serving dish and spread evenly.

Roughly chop the tomatoes, saving the juices, and spoon this evenly over the bulgar wheat. While the tomato juices are soaking in, trim and slice the spring onions finely and scatter them over the tomatoes. Finely chop the herbs and spread over the spring onions. Mix all the ingredients thoroughly.

Mix together the lemon juice, stock and allspice and pour over the tabbouleh. Toss to mix really well, season, cover, and allow the tabbouleh to stand for 30 minutes to allow the flavours to blend.

Serve with the small lettuce leaves for scooping the tabbouleh out of the dish.

Green: **Free**

HEARTY JAMBALAYA

Quorn sausages, rice and lots of vegetables combine to make a quick, yet very filling, casserole with its roots in the American Deep South.

serves 4   preparation time **20 minutes**   cooking time **25 minutes + standing time**

1 onion, peeled and finely chopped

2 red peppers, deseeded and roughly chopped

2 celery sticks, thickly sliced

2 garlic cloves, peeled and finely chopped

2 spring onions, trimmed and thinly sliced

1 tsp dried thyme

1 tsp dried oregano

3 large tomatoes

600ml/1 pint chicken stock made from Bovril

1 bay leaf

200g/7oz long grain rice

6 Quorn sausages, roughly chopped

salt and freshly ground black pepper

to garnish

chopped parsley

Place the onion, peppers, celery, garlic and spring onions in a large non-stick saucepan. Stir in the dried herbs; roughly chop the tomatoes and add to the saucepan with the chicken stock and bay leaf. Bring the mixture to the boil and add the rice and chopped Quorn sausages. Season well.

Bring back to the boil, cover very tightly, reduce the heat to low and allow to cook gently for 15–20 minutes. Remove from the heat and let sit undisturbed for 10–15 minutes.

Before serving, fluff up the grains of rice with a fork, and spoon out onto warmed plates or into bowls. Garnish with chopped parsley and serve.

EGGS

EGG, CHIP AND PEPPER BAKE

This is a really spectacular dish for a family brunch or supper – the peppers add a marvellous colour and flavour to good old egg and chips.

serves 4   preparation time **10 minutes**   cooking time **35 minutes**

1kg/2lb 4oz Desirée potatoes

Fry Light for spraying

1 red pepper, deseeded and thinly
   sliced

1 yellow pepper, deseeded and thinly
   sliced

4 large eggs

salt and freshly ground black pepper

to garnish

chopped parsley

Preheat the oven to 240°C/Gas 9. Peel the potatoes and cut them into 1cm/½in thick, long chips. Place in a saucepan of boiling water and cook for 4–5 minutes. Drain carefully and spread out onto kitchen paper to dry.

Place the chips in a shallow medium-sized ovenproof dish or four individual gratin dishes. Spray with Fry Light and bake for 10 minutes. Mix the pepper slices together and add to the potatoes and continue to bake for another 15 minutes, turning occasionally.

Remove the dish or dishes from the oven and make four wells in the chip mixture. Break an egg into each well and return to the oven for 5–6 minutes or until the eggs are cooked to your liking. Serve hot, seasoned and sprinkled with chopped parsley.

Green: **Free**

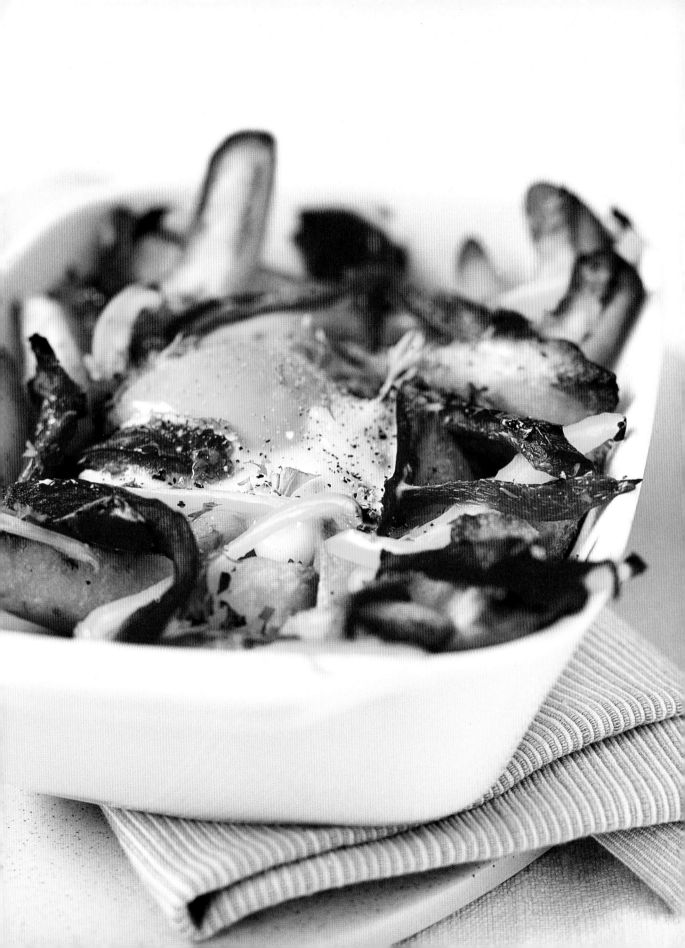

HAM, HERB AND EGG SOUFFLÉED SAVOURY CUSTARDS

Take a ham omelette a step further with these individual soufflés, which would be lovely for a light lunch served with a crisp salad.

serves 4   preparation time **10 minutes**   cooking time **12 minutes**

4 eggs, separated

1 x 200g/7oz can lean ham, finely diced

salt and freshly ground black pepper

4 tbsp very low-fat natural fromage frais

1 tsp mustard powder mixed with 2 tsp water

4 tbsp very finely chopped parsley

2 tbsp very finely chopped chives

Fry Light for spraying

Preheat the oven to 220°C/Gas 7. Place the egg yolks in a bowl and lightly beat. Add the ham to the yolk mixture and season well. Beat in the fromage frais and the mustard mixture. Stir in the herbs to mix well.

In a separate bowl, whisk the egg whites until softly peaked and then fold into the yolk mixture.

Lightly spray four individual gratin dishes or largish individual ramekin dishes with Fry Light. Divide the egg mixture between them, making sure the ham is evenly distributed between the four dishes. Place in the oven and cook for 10–12 minutes or until the mixture is slightly risen and is lightly golden on the surface. Remove from the oven and serve immediately.

Original: **Free**

CORIANDER, CHILLI AND EGG WHITE OMELETTE

Coriander and chilli add a fresh Indian tang to a tomato and onion omelette, which is substantial enough to serve cut into wedges, Spanish-omelette style.

serves 2 preparation time **10 minutes** cooking time **10 minutes**

4 egg whites

4 tbsp chopped coriander

1 red chilli, deseeded and finely sliced

1 plum tomato, deseeded and finely diced

2 spring onions, trimmed and thinly sliced

salt and freshly ground black pepper

Fry Light for spraying

Place the egg whites in a large bowl and whisk until softly peaked.

Add the coriander, chilli, tomato and spring onion to the egg white mixture, season and stir to mix well.

Spray a medium-sized non-stick frying pan with Fry Light and place over a medium heat. Pour in the egg white mixture and cook gently for 5–6 minutes. Remove from the heat and place under a medium–hot grill for 3–4 minutes or until the top is just set. Remove from the grill and serve cut into wedges.

STUFFED HERBED PANCAKE ROLLS

Half-omelette, half-pancake, this super-savoury mixture of egg with peppers and chilli, stuffed with a spicy herb filling, would be excellent on a picnic or as a supper snack.

serves 2 preparation time **15 minutes + chilling** cooking time **10 minutes**

4 eggs

2 tbsp very finely diced red pepper

1 red chilli, deseeded and very finely chopped

salt and freshly ground black pepper

Fry Light for spraying

for the stuffing

200g/7oz Quark soft cheese

1 tsp Tabasco sauce

1 tsp Worcestershire sauce

8 tbsp very finely chopped mixed fresh herbs (coriander, mint and parsley)

to serve

tomato, cucumber and mixed-leaf salad

Lightly beat the eggs with 1–2 tbsp of cold water. Stir in the diced red pepper and chilli. Season well with salt.

Spray a medium-sized non-stick frying pan with Fry Light and when hot ladle half the beaten egg mixture into it. Swirl the frying pan to coat the base evenly and cook over a gentle heat for 3–4 minutes or until the base is lightly browned and set. With a spatula, carefully slide the 'pancake' onto a clean work surface. Repeat with the remaining egg mixture to give you two pancakes. Set aside to cool.

In a bowl, mix together the Quark, Tabasco and Worcestershire sauces and the chopped mixed herbs. Season and carefully spread this mixture onto the cooled pancakes. Roll up each pancake to enclose the filling neatly and wrap each one in plastic wrap. Place in the fridge for 2–3 hours.

When ready to serve, cut the pancakes into thick diagonal slices and serve with a fresh salad of tomatoes, cucumber and mixed leaves.

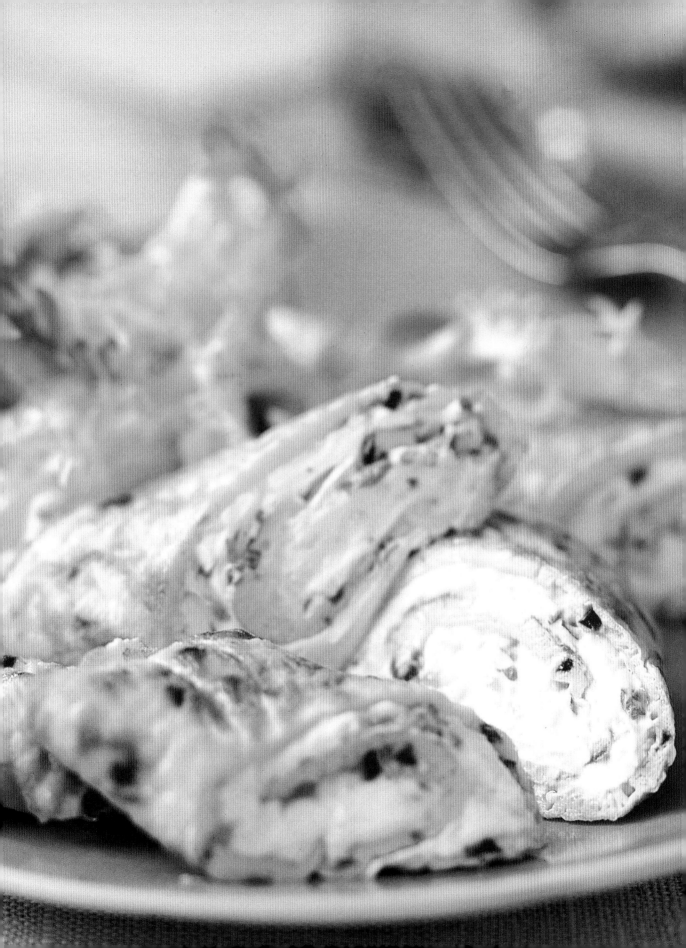

BROCCOLI, CHILLI AND PARSLEY FRITTATA

You can experiment with all kinds of fillings for a frittata, or flat, set omelette. This version uses broccoli, chilli and parsley for maximum colour and crunch.

serves 4 preparation time **15 minutes** cooking time **20 minutes**

400g/14oz broccoli, cut into small florets

Fry Light for spraying

4 spring onions, trimmed and finely sliced

1 red chilli, deseeded and finely sliced

6 eggs

4 tbsp finely chopped flat-leaf parsley

salt and freshly ground black pepper

Bring a large pan of lightly salted water to the boil and add the broccoli. Cook for 3–4 minutes and then drain thoroughly.

Spray a medium-sized non-stick frying pan with Fry Light. Add the spring onions and chilli and cook over a medium heat for 2–3 minutes. Add the drained broccoli and stir-fry for 2–3 minutes.

Beat the eggs in a bowl and stir in the chopped parsley. Season well and pour into the pan over the vegetables. Cook gently for 5–6 minutes or until the bottom of the frittata is lightly browned and set.

Place the frying pan under a medium–hot grill and cook for 5–6 minutes or until the top is just set and golden. Remove from the grill, allow to stand for 5 minutes before cutting into wedges and serving with a big crispy salad.

Green/Original **Free**

SPICED TOMATO EGGY POTATO WEDGES

This deliciously warming combination of creamy scrambled egg and spicy potato wedges would make a really filling and tasty winter supper.

serves 4   preparation time **15 minutes**   cooking time **25 minutes**

6–8 potatoes (Desirée or Maris Piper),
   cut into thick wedges
Fry Light for spraying
2 tsp paprika
1 tsp curry powder

2 tsp sea salt
8 eggs
50g/2oz very low-fat fromage frais
2 plum tomatoes, roughly chopped
salt and freshly ground black pepper

Preheat the oven to 200°C/Gas 6 and line a baking sheet with non-stick baking parchment.

Place the potatoes in a large saucepan of lightly salted boiling water for 3–4 minutes. Drain thoroughly and place on the prepared baking sheet. Spray with Fry Light. Mix together the paprika, curry powder and sea salt and sprinkle over the potato wedges. Place in the oven and bake for 15–20 minutes.

Meanwhile, beat the eggs in a bowl with the fromage frais. Stir in the tomatoes and season well. Spray a large non-stick frying pan with Fry Light and add the egg mixture. Cook over a medium heat, stirring constantly until scrambled and cooked to your liking.

Remove the wedges from the oven and divide between four warmed plates. Top each portion with the tomato eggs. Serve hot.

EGG CURRY

This egg curry is Free on both Green and Original days, so you could easily include it as part of an Indian *thali* (buffet).

serves 2   preparation time **10 minutes**   cooking time **20 minutes**

4 large eggs

Fry Light for spraying

2 small red onions, peeled and sliced

2 tbsp medium or hot curry powder

1 x 400g/14oz can chopped tomatoes

150ml/5fl oz chicken stock made
  from Bovril

salt

to serve

mild chilli powder or paprika to
  sprinkle

4 tbsp finely chopped fresh coriander
  leaves

finely chopped cucumber, tomato and
  red onion salad

Boil the eggs for 5–6 minutes and then cool and peel carefully.

Spray a large frying pan with Fry Light and place over a medium heat. Add the onion and stir-fry for 3–4 minutes. Add the curry powder and stir and cook for 1–2 minutes before adding the tomatoes and stock and seasoning with salt.

Bring the mixture to the boil, cover the pan and reduce the heat to low. Allow to cook gently for 10–12 minutes, stirring occasionally.

To serve, halve the eggs and put four halves on each plate and top with the curry sauce. Garnish with a sprinkling of chilli powder or paprika and coriander. Serve immediately with a chopped salad of cucumber, tomato and red onion.

Green/Original: **Free**

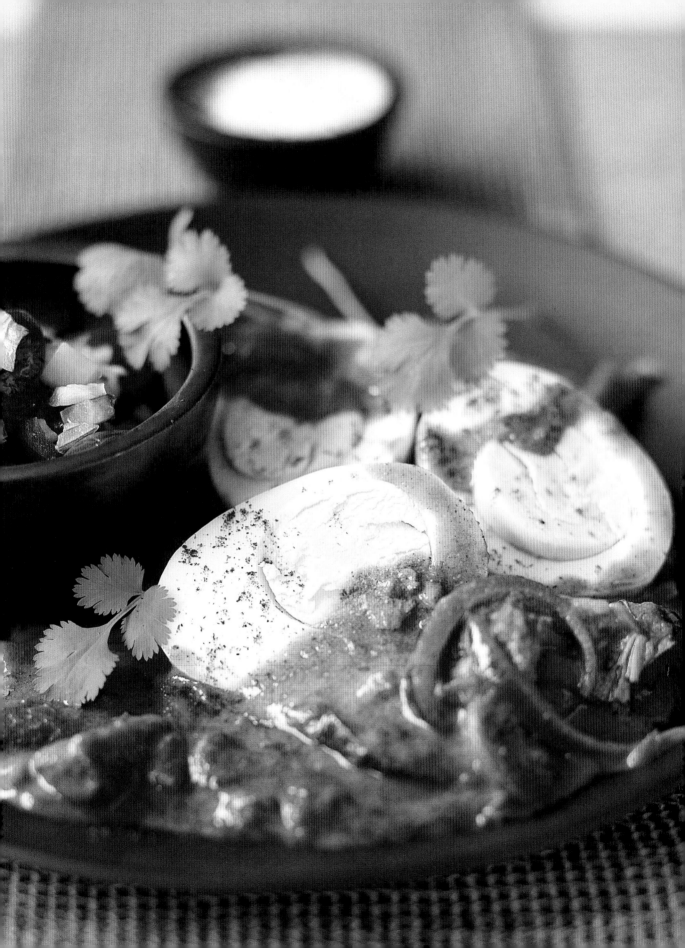

SMOKED SALMON FLORENTINE

Served on a bed of savoury spinach and topped with a softly poached egg, smoked salmon becomes even more special as a starter or supper dish.

serves 4   preparation time **15 minutes**   cooking time **10 minutes**

2 tsp white wine vinegar

4 large eggs

60ml/2fl oz chicken stock made from Bovril

500g/1lb 2oz baby leaf spinach

8 spring onions, trimmed and finely sliced

salt and freshly ground black pepper

a pinch of grated nutmeg

400g/14oz smoked salmon, sliced

Fill a deep frying pan with water and bring to the boil. Add the vinegar and reduce to a simmer. Carefully break the eggs, one at a time, into a little cup or bowl and gently slide into the simmering water. Cook for about 4–5 minutes or until cooked to your liking, then carefully remove from the pan with a slotted spoon, drain and set aside.

While the eggs are poaching, place the stock in a separate frying pan and bring to the boil. Add the spinach and spring onions, stir, cover and cook gently for 3–4 minutes or until the spinach has wilted. Season well, drain and sprinkle over the nutmeg.

Divide the spinach mixture between four warmed plates. Top with the smoked salmon slices and finish off the dish with a poached egg on top. Season and serve immediately.

SMOKED TROUT WITH ASPARAGUS-SPIKED SCRAMBLED EGGS

Smoked fish and scrambled eggs are a marriage made in heaven; this version adds lightly cooked asparagus tips for extra colour and flavour.

serves 4   preparation time **15 minutes**   cooking time **8 minutes**

100g/4oz asparagus tips

8 eggs, beaten

3 tbsp finely snipped chives

salt and freshly ground black pepper

Fry Light for spraying

2 tbsp very low-fat natural fromage
  frais

400g/14oz thinly sliced smoked trout

to garnish

lemon wedges

Bring a pan of lightly salted water to the boil, add the asparagus and cook briefly for 3–4 minutes. Drain and keep warm.

Mix the beaten eggs with the chives and season well. Spray a large non-stick frying pan with Fry Light and add the egg mixture. Cook over a medium–low heat, stirring all the time, until the eggs are scrambled to your liking. Remove from the heat and stir in the fromage frais and asparagus tips. Divide this mixture between four warmed plates and serve with the slices of smoked trout. Garnish each plate with lemon wedges.

CHICKEN, PIMENTO AND SPRING ONION EGG 'PIZZAS'

The 'pizza' base here is made from cooked egg flavoured with tasty pimento and onion; adding cooked chicken and spring onions makes a satisfying dish to eat hot or cold.

serves 2 preparation time **15 minutes** cooking time **20 minutes**

1 x 100g/4oz can pimento, drained
Fry Light for spraying
1 red onion, peeled and finely diced
4 large eggs
200g/7oz cooked chicken breast,
  skinned

4 spring onions, trimmed and finely
  sliced
salt and freshly ground black pepper

Pat the pimento dry with kitchen paper and cut into small dice. Spray a medium-sized non-stick frying pan with Fry Light. Add the onion and stir and cook over a medium heat for 3–4 minutes or until softened.

Add the chopped pimentos and stir to mix well. Spread the mixture evenly over the base of the frying pan.

Beat the eggs in a mixing bowl and pour into the frying pan. Cook gently for 4–5 minutes.

Meanwhile, tear the chicken into bite-sized strips and scatter over the egg mixture with the spring onions. Season well and cover the pan with a lid, turn the heat to low, and cook for 8–10 minutes or until the egg mixture has completely set. Remove from the heat.

To serve, cut into wedges and accompany with a large mixed salad.

BREAKFAST HASH
WITH EGGS

There's nothing better than a 'full English' breakfast and this version will set you up for whatever the day has in store – hard to believe it's Free on Original days!

serves 4   preparation time **20 minutes**   cooking time **30 minutes**

6 Quorn sausages

Fry Light for spraying

2 onions, peeled and roughly chopped

250g/9oz button mushrooms, roughly chopped

300g/11oz cherry tomatoes

6 rashers of lean bacon, trimmed of all visible fat

salt and freshly ground black pepper

4 eggs

Preheat the oven to 200°C/Gas 6. Line two baking sheets with non-stick baking parchment. On one tray place the sausages, spray with Fry Light and place in the oven.

Arrange the onions, mushrooms, cherry tomatoes and bacon on the second baking sheet, spray with Fry Light and season well. Ten minutes after the sausages have gone in, place the tray with the onions, mushrooms, cherry tomatoes and bacon in the oven and cook for 20 minutes.

Meanwhile, cook the eggs to your liking by frying them in a non-stick frying pan lightly sprayed with Fry Light. Keep warm.

Remove the sausages from the oven and roughly chop. Transfer to a bowl, remove the onion tray from the oven and add the onions, mushrooms and cherry tomatoes to the sausage mixture. Roughly chop the bacon and add to the bowl. Stir to mix well.

To serve, divide the hash mixture between four warmed plates and top each one with a fried egg.

ASPARAGUS AND HAM
OPEN EGG WHITE OMELETTE

Using egg whites for this omelette makes it extra-light and by whisking the mixture, it melts in your mouth even more easily.

serves 2 preparation time **10 minutes** cooking time **8 minutes**

100g/4oz asparagus spears

1 x 200g/7oz can lean ham

3 egg whites

2 tbsp chopped flat-leaf parsley

salt and freshly ground black pepper

Fry Light for spraying

to serve

mixed salad (optional)

Bring a large pan of lightly salted water to the boil. Trim the asparagus spears and drop in the water and blanch for 2–3 minutes until just tender. Drain and rinse under cold water. Set aside.

Chop the ham into 1cm/$\frac{1}{2}$in cubes and add to the asparagus.

Whisk the egg whites in a large bowl until softly peaked and then stir in the chopped parsley. Season well.

Spray a medium-sized non-stick frying pan with Fry Light and place over a medium heat. Pour in the egg white mixture and swirl the pan to coat the base evenly. Sprinkle over the asparagus and ham, cover and cook gently for 5–6 minutes or until the base of the omelette is just set.

Remove from the heat and serve immediately with a mixed salad, if desired.

Original: Free

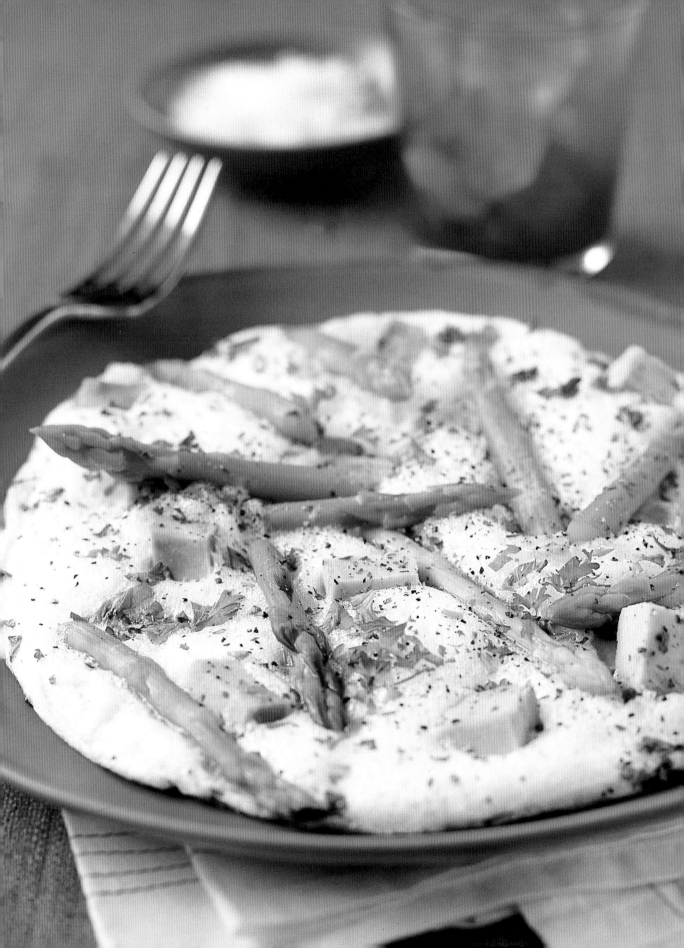

OPEN BACON AND EGG SANDWICHES

Combining the chopped egg and bacon in a creamy mustard dressing makes the ideal topping for juicy, chunky field mushrooms – fantastic for a special brunch at the weekend.

serves 4 preparation time **15 minutes** cooking time **10 minutes**

4 large flat mushrooms

Fry Light for spraying

salt and freshly ground black pepper

8 rashers of lean bacon, trimmed of all
  visible fat

4 tbsp very low-fat natural
  fromage frais

½ small shallot, very finely chopped

2 tbsp very finely chopped gherkins

1 tsp mustard powder mixed with
  2 tsp water

4 hard-boiled eggs

to garnish

a small bunch of watercress

Arrange the mushrooms on a grill rack, gill sides up, spray with Fry Light and season well. Place under a hot grill for 4–5 minutes or until just tender. Remove and set aside.

Place the bacon on the grill rack under a hot grill and cook for 4–5 minutes or until crisp. Remove and cut into bite-sized pieces. Transfer to a mixing bowl.

Add the fromage frais, shallot, gherkins and mustard mixture to the bowl and stir to mix well. Finely chop the eggs and add to this mixture. Season well.

To serve, arrange the grilled mushrooms on warmed serving plates. Top each with a few sprigs of watercress and then spoon over the bacon and egg mixture. Eat immediately.

Original Free

THAI-STYLE STUFFED DUCK EGG NETS

A 'net' is a lacy egg pancake, which in this recipe is stuffed with a Thai-style spicy rice mixture. Impressive to look at, delicious to eat – and a talking-point!

serves 4   preparation time **15 minutes**   cooking time **15 minutes**

for the stuffing

200g/7oz cooked Basmati rice

a large handful of chopped coriander

2 tbsp chopped mint leaves

1 red chilli, deseeded and finely sliced

2 spring onions, trimmed and finely
  sliced

2 tomatoes, roughly chopped

1 tbsp fish sauce

1 tsp Tabasco sauce

for the egg nets

Fry Light for spraying

4 duck eggs

salt and freshly ground black pepper

To make the stuffing, combine in a large mixing bowl the cooked rice, coriander, mint, chilli, spring onions, tomatoes, fish sauce and Tabasco. Set aside.

To make the egg nets, spray a medium-sized non-stick frying pan with Fry Light. Beat the duck eggs in a bowl and season well. Place the frying pan over a medium heat.

Working carefully and quickly, pour one quarter of the egg mixture into a piping syringe dispenser or a piping bag fitted with a single hole nozzle about 2mm/$\frac{1}{10}$in wide. Place your finger over the nozzle to stop the flow of the egg mixture and hold over the pan. Removing your finger from the nozzle, trail the egg mixture across the pan, back and forth in a zigzag to form a lacy pancake about 13cm/5in in diameter. Cook for 2–3 minutes or until the 'net' is set, then carefully remove from the pan and transfer to a plate. Repeat three more times with the remaining egg mixture to make four 'nets'.

Put a quarter of the rice mixture in the centre of each pancake, turn in the edges to make a neat parcel and serve immediately.

SALADS

FRUITY PASTA SALAD WITH ORANGES AND GRAPES

A tangy, sweet–savoury fruit salad, which goes perfectly with pasta shapes for a really refreshing and filling lunch that's full of vitamin C.

serves 4   preparation time **15 minutes**   cooking time **12 minutes**

250g/9oz dried pasta shapes

3 tbsp red wine vinegar

1 tsp English mustard powder

1 tsp artificial sweetener

salt and freshly ground pepper

150g/5oz red seedless grapes

150g/5oz green seedless grapes

2 oranges

a large bunch of chives, finely snipped

Cook the pasta according to the packet instructions, drain, transfer to a salad bowl and set aside.

Mix together the red wine vinegar with the mustard and sweetener in a small bowl. Season and mix well. Pour this mixture over the pasta and toss well to coat evenly.

Halve the grapes and add to the pasta mixture. Cut the orange into segments and add to the pasta salad. Sprinkle over the chopped chives, toss to combine and serve.

Green: **Free**

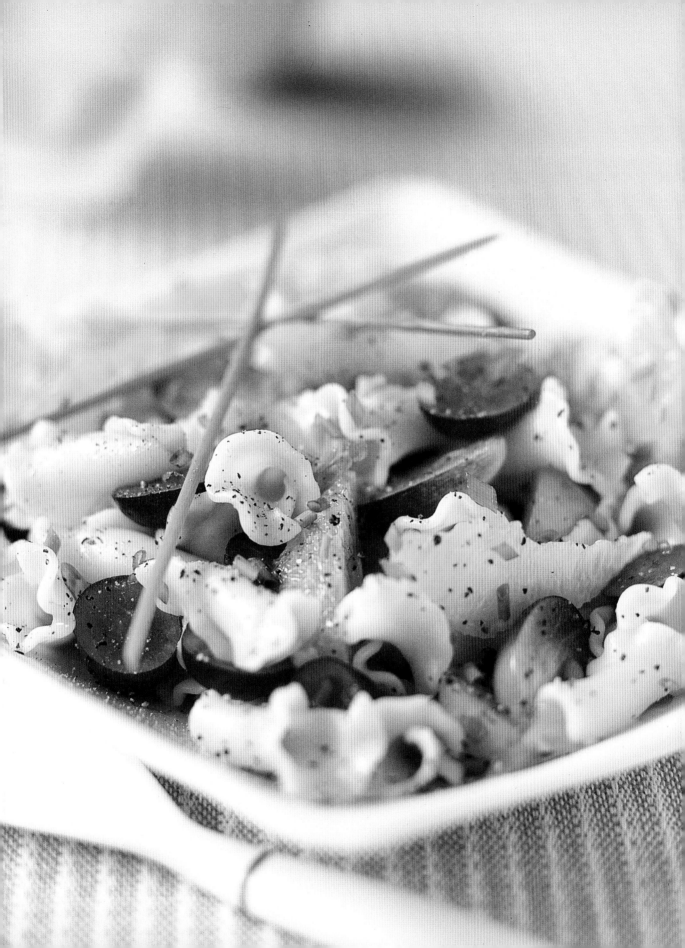

ITALIAN-STYLE TOMATO, BASIL AND CHEESE SALAD

Ripe tomatoes, vegetables and herbs create a colourful plate that makes a cottage cheese salad something special.

serves 4 preparation time **10 minutes**

8 ripe plum tomatoes

1 cucumber

1 red onion

6 tbsp finely chopped basil leaves

400g/14oz very low-fat natural cottage
   cheese

8 tbsp fat-free French-style salad
   dressing

salt and freshly ground black pepper

Using a sharp serrated knife, slice the tomatoes, cucumber and onion very thinly. Layer four serving plates with the sliced vegetables and the basil.

Divide the cottage cheese into four portions and spoon over the top of the salad. Drizzle over the salad dressing, season and serve immediately.

Green/Original: **Free**

HERBED COUSCOUS SALAD

Couscous lends itself to all kinds of different flavours; here it is teamed with a citrusy, spicy dressing, crunchy vegetables and a handful of fresh herbs.

serves 4 preparation time **15 minutes**

250g/9oz couscous

1 cucumber, finely diced

4 plum tomatoes, roughly chopped

1 red onion, peeled and finely diced

6 tbsp chopped coriander

6 tbsp chopped mint leaves

for the dressing

finely grated zest and juice of 1 lemon

1 tsp ground cumin

1 garlic clove, peeled and crushed

60ml/2fl oz chicken stock made from
  Bovril

1 red chilli, deseeded and finely sliced

salt

Place the couscous in a large bowl and pour over boiling hot water to just cover. Cover with a lid and let stand for 10–12 minutes.

Meanwhile, place the cucumber, tomatoes and onion in a large salad bowl together with the chopped herbs. Fluff up the grains of the couscous with a fork and add to the salad ingredients.

Make the dressing by mixing together the lemon zest and juice, cumin, garlic, stock and red chilli. Season with salt and stir to mix well.

Pour the dressing over the couscous salad, toss to mix well and serve at room temperature.

WILD RICE AND CARROT SALAD

Rice salad is very versatile; it travels well on picnics or in lunchboxes and is always popular at a party buffet. This recipe features the added crunch of wild rice and is full of colour as well as flavour.

serves 4 preparation time **15 minutes** cooking time **10 minutes**

200g/7oz mixed wild and Basmati rice
salt
2 carrots, peeled and cut into
 matchsticks
200g/7oz green beans, halved
 lengthways
2 ripe plum tomatoes, roughly chopped

1 red onion, peeled, halved and thinly
 sliced
200g/7oz sweetcorn niblets, rinsed and
 drained
4 tbsp fat-free French-style salad
 dressing

Cook the rice according to the packet instructions. Drain and rinse in cold water to cool. Drain again, shaking off any excess water and place the rice in a large shallow salad bowl.

Bring a large pan of lightly salted water to boil. Add the carrots and beans and cook for 3 minutes before draining and rinsing under cold water to cool. Add to the rice with the chopped tomatoes, red onion and sweetcorn.

Pour over the dressing and toss the salad ingredients to mix well. Serve immediately.

Green: **Free**

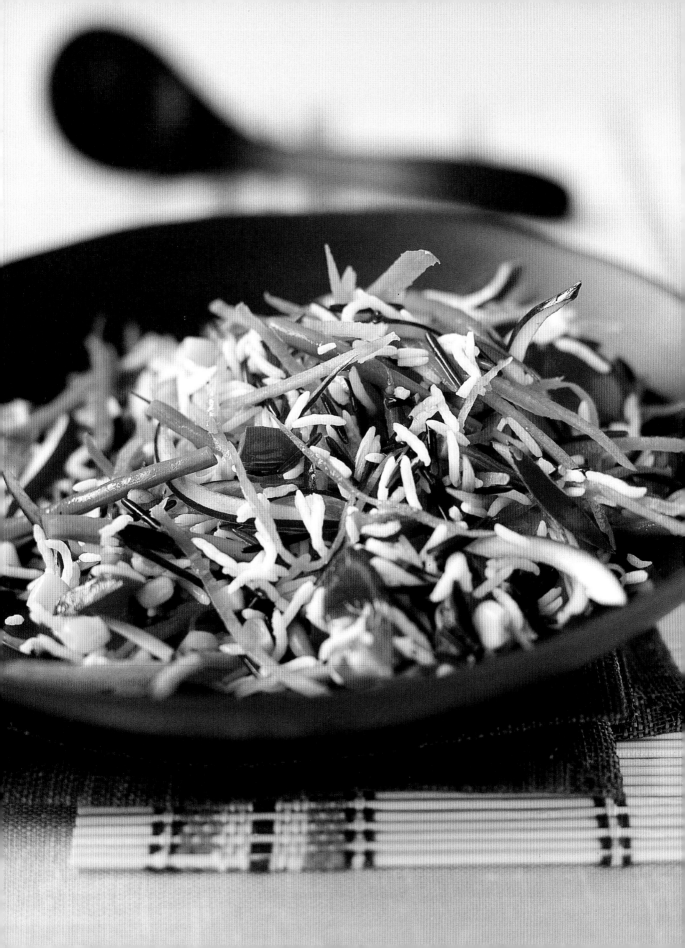

BASIL, CHILLI AND LEMON PASTA SALAD

Bold, spiky flavours of chilli and lemon are cooled with a creamy fromage frais dressing in this delicious summer pasta salad.

serves 4   preparation time **10 minutes**   cooking time **12 minutes**

250g/9oz dried farfalle or short pasta shapes

1 lemon

200g/7oz very low-fat natural fromage frais

1 tsp celery salt

8 tbsp chopped basil leaves

1 green chilli, deseeded and finely chopped

salt and freshly ground black pepper

4 spring onions, trimmed and finely sliced

Cook the pasta according to the packet instructions. Drain, rinse under cold running water, drain again and transfer to a serving bowl and set aside.

Finely grate the lemon rind into a bowl and squeeze in the juice. Add the fromage frais, celery salt, chopped basil and green chilli. Season well.

Add the spring onions to the pasta and pour in the fromage frais mixture. Toss to mix well. Serve the salad lightly chilled or at room temperature.

Green: **Free**

SPINACH AND BEANSPROUT SALAD

Ready in less than 15 minutes, this salad is a refreshing blend of fruity flavours, colours and textures with an Oriental twist.

serves 4   preparation time **10 minutes**   cooking time **3 minutes**

200g/7oz baby sweetcorn

1 x 100g/4oz bag fresh baby spinach
   leaves

½ small pineapple

100g/4oz beansprouts

1 x 200g/7oz can water chestnuts,
   drained

for the dressing

4 tbsp light soy sauce

juice of 1 lime

30ml/1fl oz chicken stock made from
   Bovril

3 tbsp chopped coriander

Bring a saucepan of water to the boil. Add the baby sweetcorn and cook for 2–3 minutes. Drain and refresh under cold water and drain again. Transfer to a mixing bowl with the spinach leaves.

Peel, core and cut the pineapple into bite-sized pieces. Add to the salad bowl with the beansprouts and water chestnuts.

Make the dressing by mixing together the soy sauce, lime juice, chicken stock and coriander in a bowl. Pour over the salad ingredients and toss to mix well. Divide the salad into four large bowls and serve.

MINTED TROPICAL FRUIT SALAD

The perfect end to a meal, a tropical fruit salad spiked with mint is super-healthy, very refreshing and is easily made in advance and left to chill.

serves 4   preparation time **25 minutes**

3 ripe mangoes

8 large kiwi fruit

1/2 small green melon

1 small honeydew melon

250g/9oz watermelon wedge, seeds removed

to serve

a handful of fresh mint leaves

Cut the cheeks off the sides of the mangoes and, using a melon baller, make balls of the mango flesh and place in a bowl. Cut the kiwi fruit in half and, using the melon baller again, repeat and add the kiwi balls to the mangoes. Halve the melon and deseed. Repeat the procedure with the melon baller to give you melon and watermelon balls.

Divide the mixed fruit balls between four dessert bowls and scatter over the mint leaves. Serve chilled.

Green/Original: **Free**

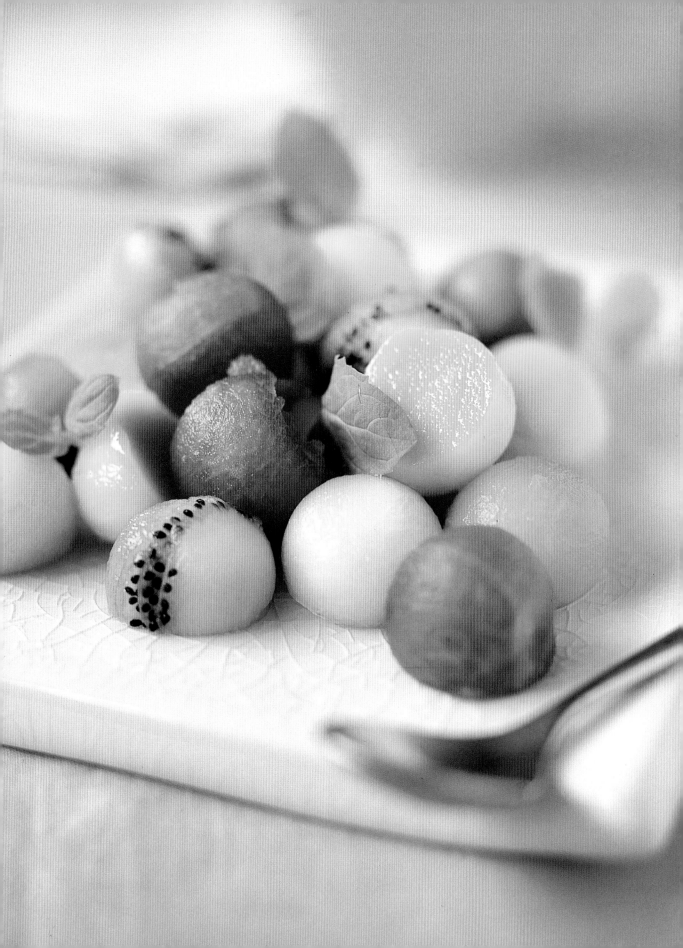

BABY ROASTED POTATO AND MIXED GREENS SALAD

Combining roasted potatoes with sugar snap peas and a mildly spiced yogurt dressing gives an intriguing twist to the ever-popular potato salad.

serves 4   preparation time **15 minutes**   cooking time **25 minutes**

700g/1lb 9oz baby new potatoes
salt and freshly ground black pepper
Fry Light for spraying
400g/14oz sugar snap peas
50g/2oz mixed salad leaves

for the dressing
1 tsp roasted cumin seeds
I tsp ground coriander
juice of 1 lemon
200g/7oz very low-fat natural yogurt
60ml/2fl oz chicken stock made from Bovril

Preheat the oven to 220°C/Gas 7. Place the potatoes on a non-stick baking tray and season well. Spray with Fry Light and roast in the oven for 20–25 minutes or until tender. Set aside to cool.

Meanwhile, halve the sugar snap peas, place in lightly salted boiling water and boil for 2–3 minutes. Drain and refresh under cold running water, drain again and transfer to a bowl.

Make the dressing by mixing together all the ingredients and season well.

To serve, mix the potatoes and sugar snap peas together. Divide the salad leaves between four plates and top with the roasted potato and sugar snap mixture. Drizzle the dressing over the top of the salads and serve immediately.

Green: **Free**

ALL-DAY BREAKFAST SALAD

Can't decide whether to have a cooked breakfast or a salad? Have both – with a clever recipe that creates a substantial, tasty meal at any time of day.

serves 4   preparation time **15 minutes**   cooking time **15 minutes**

Fry Light for spraying

250g/9oz baby button mushrooms, halved

12 rashers of lean bacon, trimmed of all visible fat

4 plum tomatoes

2 baby gem lettuce

4 hard-boiled eggs

3 tbsp chopped chives

for the dressing

100g/4oz very low-fat natural fromage frais

100ml/3½fl oz passata

1 tsp mustard powder mixed with 2 tsp water

salt and freshly ground black pepper

Spray a large non-stick frying pan with Fry Light and add the mushrooms and cook over a high heat for 3–4 minutes or until the mushrooms are tender and lightly browned. Transfer to a salad bowl.

Add the bacon to the frying pan and cook for 3–4 minutes on each side or until crisp and lightly browned. Drain on kitchen paper, then cut into bite-sized pieces and add to the mushrooms.

Cut the tomatoes into wedges, roughly tear the lettuce leaves and add to the salad ingredients. Roughly chop the eggs and sprinkle on top of the salad ingredients and then add the chives.

Make the dressing by mixing together all the ingredients in a bowl.

To serve, divide the salad mixture between four plates and drizzle over the dressing.

ROASTED BEETROOT AND CORIANDER SALAD

A beautiful red and green salad that tastes as good as it looks, dressed with a refreshing blend of mild spices and natural yogurt.

serves 4   preparation time **10 minutes**   cooking time **45 minutes**

750g/1lb 10oz beetroot
Fry Light for spraying
400g/14oz runner beans
100g/4oz wild rocket leaves

for the dressing
1 tsp ground coriander
1 tsp ground cumin
2 tbsp very finely chopped fresh
   coriander
200g/7oz very low-fat natural yogurt
salt and freshly ground black pepper

Preheat the oven to 220°C/Gas 7. Place the beetroot on a baking sheet and lightly spray with Fry Light. Roast in the oven for 35–40 minutes or until cooked and just tender. Remove from the oven and allow to cool before peeling off the skin and cutting into thick slices or bite-sized pieces. Transfer to a bowl and set aside.

Meanwhile, slice the runner beans diagonally and blanch for 2–3 minutes in a large saucepan of lightly salted boiling water. Drain and rinse under cold running water and drain again. Add to the beetroot.

Make the dressing by mixing together the ground spices, coriander, yogurt and 60ml/2fl oz water. Season.

To serve the salad, divide the beetroot mixture between four serving plates and add the rocket leaves. Drizzle over the dressing and serve immediately.

Green/Original: **Free**

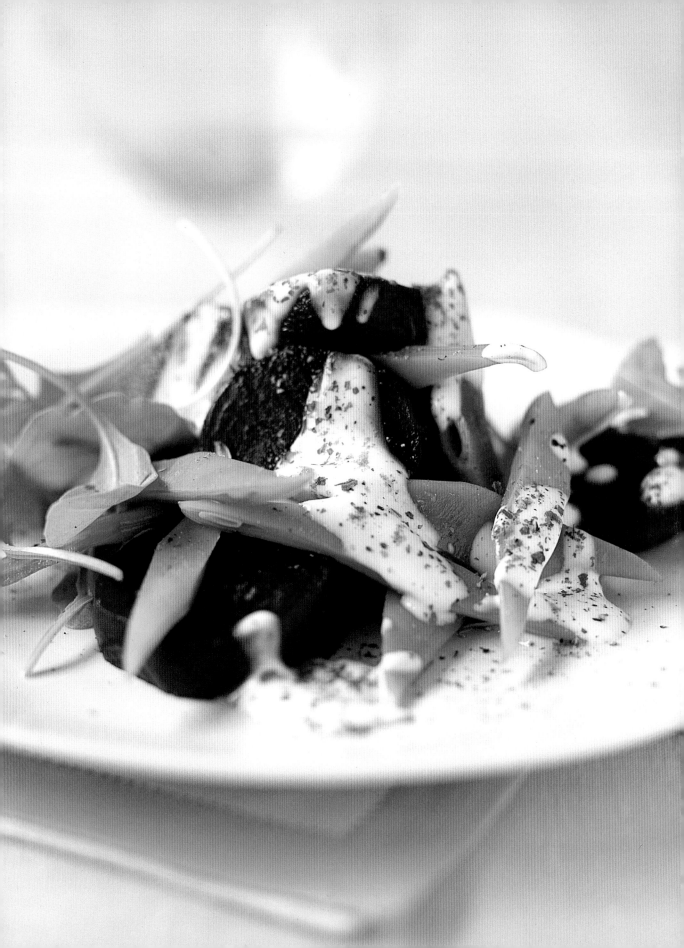

GREEN BEAN
AND LENTIL SALAD

Lentils work just as well cold in salads as they do in stews and soups. Here, their flavour is enhanced with flat-leaf parsley and a fat-free salad dressing.

serves 4 preparation time **15 minutes** cooking time **25 minutes**

150g/5oz puy lentils

400g/14oz green beans

1 carrot

2 celery sticks

4 plum tomatoes

2 shallots, peeled

a large handful of roughly chopped
 flat-leaf parsley

6 tbsp fat-free French-style salad
 dressing

salt and freshly ground black pepper

Rinse the lentils, drain and place in a large saucepan. Fill the saucepan with cold water and bring to the boil. Cook for 20–25 minutes and then drain. Rinse under cold water, drain and set aside.

While the lentils are cooking, trim the green beans and cut into 2.5cm/1in lengths. Blanch in boiling water for 1 minute, then drain and leave to cool. Peel and cut the carrot into fine dice and place them in a saucepan of boiling water and boil for 5–6 minutes. Drain and cool.

Finely slice the celery and place in a bowl. Add the lentils, beans and carrots. Roughly chop the tomatoes, finely chop the shallots and add to the bean mixture with the parsley. Stir in the dressing and toss to mix well. Season and serve at room temperature.

Green: **Free**

SUMMER PRAWN SALAD

A big bowl of this colourful salad would be perfect to dip into as part of a lazy summer lunch – and it only takes 15 minutes to put together.

serves 4   preparation time **15 minutes**

800g/1lb 12oz cooked tiger prawns
1 large cucumber
350g/12oz cherry tomatoes
6 spring onions
25g/1oz wild rocket leaves

for the dressing
100g/4oz very low-fat natural yogurt
100g/4oz very low-fat natural
 fromage frais
8 tbsp chopped fresh dill
1 tsp artificial sweetener
juice of 1 lemon
salt and freshly ground black pepper

Place the prawns in a large mixing bowl. Peel the cucumber and then halve lengthways. Using a small spoon, deseed both the halves and discard. Cut the cucumber into thin slices and place with the prawns.

Halve the cherry tomatoes and thinly slice the spring onions and add to the salad bowl with the rocket leaves. Toss to mix well.

Make the dressing by mixing together the yogurt and fromage frais until smooth. Add the dill, sweetener and lemon juice. Season and stir to mix well.

To serve, divide the salad between four chilled plates and spoon over the dill and yogurt dressing.

TUNA, CAPERS AND MIXED GRILLED PEPPER SALAD

Capers have a uniquely tangy taste that brings out the flavour in other ingredients – in this case, a super-healthy salad of tuna and roasted mixed peppers that's easily made in advance.

serves 4 preparation time **10 minutes** cooking time **10–12 minutes**

8 mixed peppers (red, orange and
  yellow)

1 red onion

1 garlic clove, peeled and finely grated

juice of 1 lemon

2 x 200g/7oz cans tuna in brine,
  drained

3 tbsp capers or caperberries

1/2 small cucumber, cut into thin strips

salt and freshly ground black pepper

to serve

100g/4oz bag of wild rocket leaves

Halve and deseed the peppers, place them skin side up under a hot grill and cook for 10–12 minutes until the skin is blackened and charred. Remove and place in a plastic bag for 10–12 minutes. When cool, peel and cut into strips and place in a bowl with any saved juices from them.

Halve the onion, peel and thinly slice and add to the peppers with the garlic and lemon juice.

Flake the tuna into large chunks and add to the pepper mixture with the capers and cucumber. Season well and toss to mix. To serve, divide the rocket leaves between four plates and top with the tuna mixture.

Original: Free

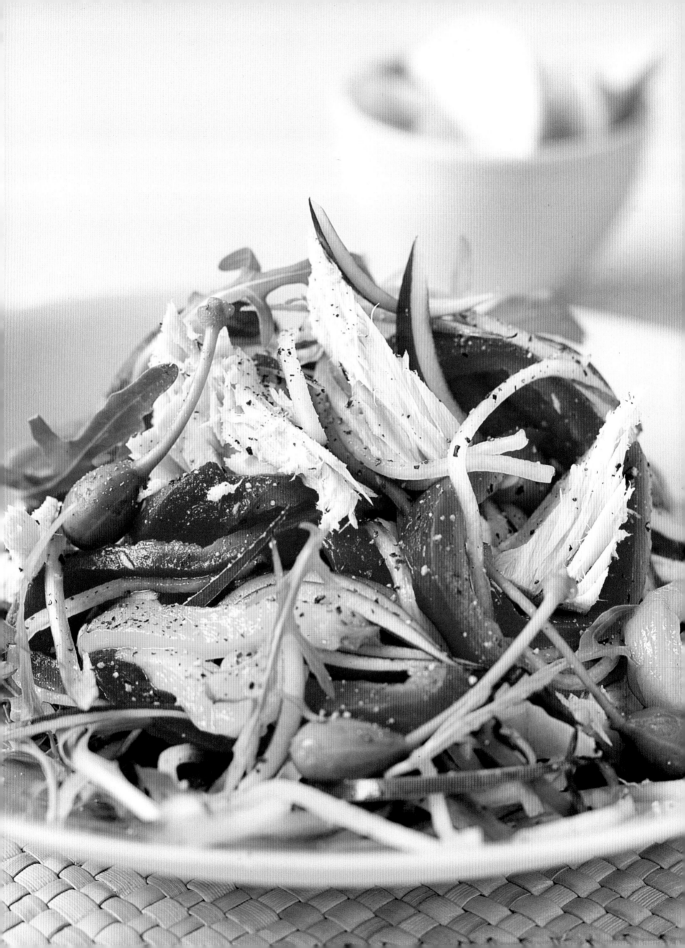

DUCK, MANGO AND WATERCRESS SALAD

Peppery watercress, sweet mango, rich duck breast and crunchy red pepper combine in a luxurious salad with a tropical, Oriental tang.

serves 4 preparation time **15 minutes** cooking time **16 minutes**

4 skinless duck breasts, trimmed of all
   visible fat
salt and freshly ground black pepper
Fry Light for spraying
2 ripe sweet mangoes
4 spring onions, trimmed and shredded
1 red pepper, deseeded and very thinly
   sliced
a large bunch of watercress

for the dressing
4 tbsp light soy sauce
1 tsp Chinese five-spice powder
1 tbsp Worcestershire sauce
1 tsp Tabasco sauce
60ml/2fl oz chicken stock made from
   Bovril

Season the duck breasts well and spray with Fry Light. Place on a grill rack under a medium–hot grill and cook for 6–8 minutes on each side or until cooked to your liking. Remove from the grill, cover with foil and allow to rest for 10 minutes.

Meanwhile, peel, stone and cut the mangoes into bite-sized cubes and place in a large bowl with the spring onions, red pepper and watercress. Toss to mix well.

To serve, divide the salad mixture between four serving plates. Thinly slice the duck and place on top of the salad. Mix together all the dressing ingredients and serve the salad with the dressing spooned over.

Original: **Free**

PEPPERED FILLET STEAK SALAD

Juicy strips of warm fillet steak, with a touch of heat from black pepper, make the perfect partner for a simple salad of green leaves, onions and mushrooms – a brilliant new twist on an old favourite.

serves 4 preparation time **15 minutes** cooking time **10 minutes**

700g/1lb 9oz fillet steaks, trimmed of
 all visible fat
freshly ground black pepper
Fry Light for spraying
300g/11oz button mushrooms

2 x 100g/4oz bags mixed salad leaves
2 shallots, peeled and halved
 lengthways
6 tbsp fat-free vinaigrette-style dressing

Place the steaks on a clean work surface and season liberally with freshly ground black pepper. Spray them with Fry Light.

Heat a large non-stick griddle pan on a high heat and then add the steaks and cook for 3–4 minutes on each side or until cooked to your liking. Transfer to a clean work surface, cover with foil and allow to rest for 10 minutes.

While the meat is resting, wipe the mushrooms clean and thinly slice. Place in a large salad bowl with the mixed salad leaves. Thinly slice the shallots and add to the bowl. Add the salad dressing and toss to mix well.

Using a sharp serrated knife, slice the fillet steaks into thin strips.

To serve, divide the salad mixture between four large serving plates and top with the peppered fillet. Serve immediately.

FREE FOODS SELECTION

We have listed many of our Free Foods here. For the full list, you will need to become a Slimming World member.

■ Foods marked with an **S** symbol **will give your weight loss a boost**. Choosing foods marked with an **SS** symbol will give your weight loss an even **bigger boost**.

■ Foods marked with an **F** will give you **extra fibre** and those marked with **FF** will give you an even **richer helping of fibre**.

■ Foods marked **H** will keep you **healthy** and those marked **HH** are **vital to your health** and need to be included in your diet **every day**.

S	weight loss boost
SS	extra weight loss boost
F	extra fibre
FF	extra-rich fibre
H	healthy
HH	vital to health

GREEN CHOICE FREE FOODS

All vegetables are classed as a Free Food when on a Green day.

Potatoes			HH
Rice			H
Dried pasta			H
Buckwheat			H
Couscous			H
Baked beans	F	SS	H
Chickpeas	F		H
Red kidney beans	FF	S	H
Soya beans	FF		H
Lentils	F	S	H
Peas	F	SS	H
Quorn	F	SS	H
Tofu			
Dairy			
Eggs			
Very low-fat natural yogurt			H
Very low-fat natural fromage frais			H
Very low-fat natural cottage cheese			H

The following fruits can be eaten freely as long as they are fresh or frozen varieties.

Apples	S	HH
Bananas		HH
Grapefruit	SS	HH
Oranges	S	HH
Peaches	S	HH
Pineapple	S	HH
Strawberries	SS	HH

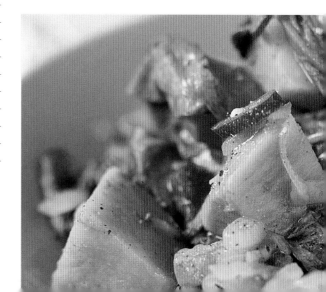

ORIGINAL CHOICE FREE FOODS

Not all vegetables are Free Foods on the Original Choice. Choose freely from the following list:

Artichokes	F	S	HH
Asparagus		S	HH
Aubergine		S	HH
Baby whole sweetcorn		S	HH
Beans – French, runner	F	S	HH
Beetroot		S	HH
Broccoli	F	S	HH
Brussels sprouts	F	S	HH
Cabbage		S	HH
Carrots		S	HH
Cauliflower		S	HH
Courgettes		S	HH
Leeks		S	HH
Mushrooms		S	HH
Onions		S	HH
Spinach		S	HH
Squash		S	HH
Swede		S	HH
Quorn	F	SS	H
Tofu			

Poultry

Chicken, no fat or skin		S	H
Turkey, no fat or skin		S	H

Meat

Bacon			
Beef			
Ham			
Lamb			
Pork			

Fish

Cod		SS	H
Haddock		SS	H
Kippers			H
Mackerel (not smoked)			H
Pilchards			H
Plaice		SS	H
Salmon (fresh, canned and smoked)			H
Sole		SS	H

Shellfish

Crab			H
Prawns		S	H
Caviare		SS	H

Dairy

Eggs			
Very low-fat natural yogurt			H
Very low-fat natural fromage frais			H
Very low-fat natrual cottage cheese			H

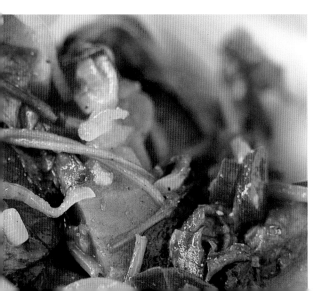

The following fruits can be eaten freely as long as they are fresh or frozen varieties.

Apples	S	HH
Bananas		HH
Grapefruit	SS	HH
Oranges	S	HH
Peaches	S	HH
Pineapple	S	HH
Strawberries	SS	HH

SYNS SELECTION

Listed below are a selection of Syn values for foods that you can enjoy every day. The values apply to both the Green and Original choices.

ALCOHOL

25ml/1fl oz measure of any spirit	2½
150ml/¼ pt glass of wine	5
300ml/½ pt lager/beer	5
300ml/½ pt cider	5

BISCUITS AND BARS Each

Cheese thin	1
Chocolate finger	1½
Rich tea/marie	2
Jaffa cake/ginger nut	2½
Shortcake	2½
Custard cream	3
Go Ahead Crispy Fruit Slices	3
Digestive	3½
Jammie Dodger	4
Special K Cereal Bar	4½

CAKES Per cake, average

Chocolate mini roll	5½
McVitie's Golden Syrup Cake Bar	6½
Mr Kipling Almond/Lemon Slices	6½
Toffee Crisp Biscuit Bar	6½
Mr Kipling Mini Battenburg	7
Mr Kipling Angel/Chocolate Slices	7½

CHOCOLATE AND SWEETS

Per standard bar/tube/bag unless stated

Milky Bar	3½
Fun-size bars	5
Two-finger Kit Kat	5½
Milky Way	6
Fudge/Curly Wurly	6½
Penguin bar	7
Polo mints	7
Maltesers	9
Flake	9

CRISPS Per standard bag

French Fries/Golden Lights	4½
Thai Bites	4½
Quavers	5
Wotsits	5½
Special K Lite Bites	6
Snack-a-Jacks	7
Standard potato crisps, per 25g/1oz	7½

DESSERTS Per pot

Müllerlight Fruit Halo	4
Müllerice, Only 1% Fat	6
Danone Goodies Strawberry Trifle	7
Müllerlight Mousse	7½

ICE CREAMS/LOLLIES

Mini Cornetto/Calippo	3
50g/2oz scoop low fat ice cream	4
Fab Ice Lolly	4
Solero	5
Strawberry Split Ice	6½
Mini Yorkie Ice Cream Bar	7

NUTS (per 25g/1oz)

Cashew nuts, shelled	8
Peanuts/almonds, fresh/roasted	8½
Brazil nuts, shelled	9½
Walnuts, shelled	10

SAUCES AND SPREADS

Custard made with skimmed milk: 2 level tbsp	1
Gravy made with no fat: 4 level tbsp	1
Reduced calorie mayonnaise: 1 level tbsp	2½
Margarine/spread low fat variety: 25g/1oz	5½
Oil/any variety: 1 level tbsp	6

INDEX